Reflexology

The Absolute Beginner's Guide to Reflexology

(Learn How to Use Reflexology With Easy Techniques and Simple Instruction)

Shawn Underwood

Published By **Cathy Nedrow**

Shawn Underwood

Reflexology: The Absolute Beginner's Guide to Reflexology (Learn How to Use Reflexology With Easy Techniques and Simple Instruction)

ISBN 978-0-9938301-1-2

No part of this guidebook shall be reproduced in any form without permission in writing from the publisher except in the case of brief quotations embodied in critical articles or reviews.

Legal & Disclaimer

The information contained in this book is not designed to replace or take the place of any form of medicine or professional medical advice. The information in this book has been provided for educational & entertainment purposes only.

The information contained in this book has been compiled from sources deemed reliable, and it is accurate to the best of the Author's knowledge; however, the Author cannot guarantee its accuracy and validity and cannot be held liable for any errors or omissions. Changes are periodically made to this book. You must consult your doctor or get professional medical advice before using any of the suggested remedies, techniques, or information in this book.

Table Of Contents

Chapter 1: What Is Reflexology?

Most parents enjoy nauseated at the same time as we keep in mind our ft. Most people keep in thoughts our toes unattractive, smelly appendages at the cease of our legs that flaunt nasty brittle nails, hard calluses, and unneeded toe hair. There's no denying that ft are top notch for purchasing us round and look amazingly blanketed up through a couple of Manolo Blahniks, but it virtually is all we're capable to say for them.

However, an more and more famous remedy focuses almost absolutely at the feet and is not handiest for kooky foot fetishists. Reflexology is touted as a simple massage that focuses totally on the toes and may cope with many conditions throughout the whole frame. Whether it truly works or no longer is, of path, every different depend.

Reflexology is a shape of bodywork based totally totally on the concept that human beings have so-known as "reflex zones" on our feet, palms, or even ears (see beneath). These regions or zones healthy distinct portions of our body. Traditionally recognized widely speakme as region therapy, reflexology has been practiced for hundreds of years, particularly with the useful resource of ancient Egyptians and Chinese.

There are 11 great bodily zones. When a reflexologist applies pressure to the ft, nerves in the toes carry calming impulses to the critical worried device, developing a experience of calm and relieving anxiety. It is idea that the paths through the spots strolling, and plenty of others., are connected to fantastic frame factors via the applicable fearful tool, that is why it allegedly works.

Therefore, the healing impact is transmitted a few other region at the same time as we push or comply with specialized pressure to tremendous zones in the hand or foot. If you have got a trouble along with your pituitary gland, you first-class want to massage your big ft, which correlate to that gland. Then voilanow not a hassle!

Dr. William H. Fitzgerald, an ear, nostril, and throat professional, and Dr. Edwin Bowers, who invented "place remedy" in 1915, contributed to the evolution of contemporary reflexology to meet our dreams. They hypothesized that the use of pressure to positive body regions need to bring about anesthetic effects on different body parts.

In the 1930s, Eunice Ingham, a physiotherapist and nurse persisted and improved their art work through reworking zone treatment into reflexology. She concept that the feet have been the maximum sensitive quantities of the body in phrases of region remedy and devised reflexology charts depicting the body regarding our little toesies (and tootsies).

Ear Reflexology.

Some people currently have interaction in ear reflexology, from time to time known as "auricular treatment." According to TCM or traditional Chinese remedy, there are spots at the ears which might be believed to hook up with the coronary heart, and it is believed that stroking these elements will ease fear and sell calmness. Other frame regions can be tormented by rubbing distinct ear components.

The ear as a window into one's health has fascinated people for ages, if now not millennia. People reportedly burned portions in their ears to ease all over again pain approximately 4 hundred BC, and auricular acupuncture acquired popularity in four hundred AD.

In the 1950s, a French scientific physician named Dr. Paul Nogier purportedly advanced the present day-day reflux mapping of ear remedy after treating sufferers who had suffered ear burns while looking to treatment high-quality ailments.

You can now workout recuperation ear rubdown for your very personal via softly caressing your ear collectively together along with your thumb and fingertip. For first-class results, a professional ear reflexologist is normally encouraged to educate you first. Avoid embarrassment with the aid of making sure you've got used a Q-tip within the ultimate 12 months or . Happy rubbing!

Reflexology is maximum of the maximum well-known opportunity remedies, and its advocates declare it presents big and lengthy-lasting health benefits. Reflexologists assert that their treatment may additionally moreover address a large form of situations, from urinary tract infections to arthritis (with the useful resource of stimulating the adrenal glands and lowering cortisone reliance) through the bladder and kidney reflex elements under the foot (by manner of taking walks the bladder and kidney factors positioned on the lowest of your foot).

However, its critics claim that it is a load of antique hogwash and that the most effective health benefit is one which anybody would possibly accumulate from spending time in a non violent, silent room whilst (preferably) receiving a fulfilling rubdown.

For example, Dr. Stephen Barrett, MD, has authored a piece of writing for QuackWatch regarding reflexology wherein he describes severa treatments he underwent to decide their effectiveness.

A reflexologist confident him that he may additionally additionally need to alleviate his excessive shoulder ache, which have been criminal for essential surgical operation, in a few periods after great one session. "His 'treatment,' which lasted approximately 10 mins, consisted of rubbing the foot and, at instances, utilizing excessive stress to the ball of my foot," Dr. Barrett wrote. "

The "treatment" did truely nothing to assist my shoulder. A few months later, I had surgical operation that right now and completely corrected the condition."

If reflexology makes you enjoy better and experience the enjoy, it may be actually really worth attempting. However, you have to see a systematic professional earlier than attempting any opportunity remedy, although it appears innocent.

Avoid this remedy if you have a foot fracture, an open foot wound, or active foot gout. Similarly, patients with lively thrombosis or embolism are affected. Consult your medical doctor first in case you are experiencing foot or leg vascular problems. Inform your reflexologist if you are in the early levels of pregnancy in order that he or she may be able to regulate your remedy as a end result.

Chapter 2: Reflexology Theories And Principles.

In conjunction with osteopathy, acupuncture, or mild treatment, reflexology has been mounted to be a as an opportunity a hit possibility treatment. It is an incredibly calming rub down approach that goals particular "reflex factors/regions" inside the toes, fingers, and ears.

These factors correlate to everyone organ, gland, and machine and are related to them via way of "zones," "energy channels," and "meridians." Energy channels grow to be clogged even as an imbalance or infection exists in the frame. Reflexology remedy techniques put off those obstructions and repair the unfastened go along with the waft of strength.

Reflexology, that is known as a holistic and healing art work, normally produces the best results whilst the practitioner works with passion and self belief. Not best does it lower muscular anxiety and pressure, but it additionally cleanses the body of dangerous impurities and pollution. Reflexology is taken into consideration "Preventative Healthcare" because it revitalizes power and restores systemic stability.

Research executed the world over indicates that reflexology blessings superb illnesses. The National Cancer Institute undertook an lousy lot research, and the National Institutes of Health determined out that reflexology can also want to reduce/lessen pain, tension, anxiety, and despair and enhance sleep, herbal recovery, and rest.

Sir Charles Sherrington and Sir Henry Head confirmed inside the Nineties that there's a neurological relationship most of the skin and internal organs and that the frame's hectic tool can adapt to a stimulus, laying the muse for the principle that reflexology works with the valuable worried tool of the body.

Therefore, regular with this concept, making use of stress to the palms, toes, or ears will transmit enjoyable and calming messages to severa body sections thru the peripheral nerves in the arms, ft, and ears.

Also, "The Gate Theory" and "The Neuromatrix Theory" deliver an explanation for why reflexology offers ache and stress remedy. The theories declare that the thoughts generates subjective ache in reaction to cognitive or emotional variables; as a give up result, emotions and times which incorporates pressure and tension can impact our perceptions of ache. Therefore, reflexology remedy alleviates pain by way of way of enhancing temper and decreasing tension.

According to each different view, the human frame possesses "essential electricity," and congestion or suffocation of the energy flow produces contamination and ailments inside the body.

Reflexology allows the motion of electricity. The "Zone Theory" divides the human frame into 10 vertical zones much like the feet and fingers as a great deal as the pinnacle.

According to this hypothesis, every muscle organ and gland in 1 / 4 is offered thru a reflex aspect on the ft or arms.

The following tenets manual the exercising of reflexology:

Practitioners do no longer heal sufferers; the body heals and fixes itself.

The practitioner isn't the healer but truely a participant.

The human frame responds to physical contact, which promotes recuperation.

Both the patron and the practitioner may also "experience" the movement of power from reflex spots on the ft, palms, and ears to different frame areas.

Reflexology can not alternative for hospital therapy

Reflexology is implemented as an opportunity or complementary treatment.

Reflexology is numerous to a foot rubdown.

According to reflexologists, maximum fitness problems are related to pressure and tension.

This is enough evidence for harassed and chronically ill humans to try this ancient remedy practiced in India, China, Egypt, and special historic civilizations. Stress-related issues, aches, pains, and mild illnesses can be dealt with with reflexology.

Chapter 3: Benefits Of Reflexology.

Reflexology is the recuperation stimulation of the ft. This is completed through utilising strain to precise foot factors. It is an historical shape of acupressure dating again lots of years. Asia has written proof of acupressure rub down practices dating all over again to 5000 BCE. Egyptian hieroglyphs referencing foot reflexology have been exposed.

Native Americans have diagnosed the connection the various foot and the whole frame for millennia. Native Americans may rub down dust and particular herbs into the soles of their feet. They utilized this approach to cope with disease, pain, and illnesses. They believed this method ought to beautify someone's fitness and repair his spirit to the Earth.

Physiological and Psychological advantages.

There are each mental and physiological advantages to reflexology. Reflexology strategies are executed by using way of making use of physical pressure to the arms and ft. This is finished with the finger, thumb, and severa hand strategies. It is considered that those strategies should now not contain the usage of components which encompass creams, creams, and oils.

Throughout data, it is been claimed that those techniques can result in a specific alteration in someone's thoughts and/or frame even as unique programs are used to govern those strategies. Here, you'll examine the physiological and intellectual advantages of reflexology.

Benefits of Physiological Reflexology:

Reflexology is assumed to reinforce the effectiveness of what is known as the "baroreceptor reflex" inside the body. This is taken into consideration certainly one of reflexology's maximum huge physiological outcomes. This "reflex" within the body has tremendous talents and obligations.

First, it's miles one of the fundamental additives of the human frame. For instance, it is one of the primary components of the body's natural homeostasis or "balance." Reflexology stimulates the body's baroreceptor reaction, enhancing blood strain regulation and comparable bodily features.

Reflexology has been located to be of super fee to people with brilliant blood go with the flow and accompanying problems. Effective blood glide is vital for organs in the course of the frame to get keep of the vitamins required for proper feature, healthful mobile renovation and manufacturing, and an growth inside the immune gadget's natural electricity and functionality to combat in competition to infectious sellers and headaches to the body can be uncovered.

Reflexology Psychological benefits:

Many intellectual blessings accrue to folks who participate in reflexology. It is alleged, for instance, that this method lets in human beings with sleep troubles, collectively with insomnia, to set up a level of relaxation that allows them to triumph over the headaches connected with this infection.

Those with chronic fatigue syndrome, lupus, or fibromyalgia also can gain from this approach, as it could help the body in overcoming sensations of weariness and resting nice whilst crucial for the top-fine functioning of the mind and frame.

Most people who be afflicted by unhealthful strain, excessive ranges of worry, or even melancholy-associated problems can experience the soothing techniques associated with reflexology.

It is concept that the physiological advantages of stepped forward blood flow and regulation, optimizing oxygen tiers inside the frame, and the calming feelings related to this approach hold the treatment for highbrow disturbances and headaches which includes tension, melancholy, and similar conditions.

Your reflexology session will begin with a slight foot "heat-up." After finishing this step, the reflexologist will exercise stress to unique locations for your foot. To stimulate the nerve finishing at the pressure net web page. The associated organ or gland will then be stimulated. Occasionally, a "crystal deposit" is determined at a selected internet web web page.

It is hypothesized that the ones crystals avoid nerve endings. Your reflexologist will use stress and massage to break up those deposits. This will create a pathway among the nerve terminal and its related organ.

How each man or woman's body responds to reflexology is particular. Some humans will see and enjoy the results as an alternative right away. Others would require more than one lessons to start noticing the preferred consequences.

As with all kinds of treatment, it is contingent upon the length and severity of the ailment. Reflexology is a complete remedy and a likely opportunity for some drug remedies. The notion that reflexology works are also important to exceptional effects. The mind-frame hyperlink is powerful; your body will respond favorably if you have a extraordinary highbrow thoughts-set.

Here are a number of the results my clients have stated to me:

Most human beings enjoy comfort from constipation inside 3 to 20-4 hours.

Cramp consolation with menstruation.

Reflexology presents strain comfort and is notably calming.

Sleeping higher and longer at night time time.

Reduced again ache.

Eradication of migraine migraines.

Reflexology, like rub down remedy, is a holistic technique to recovery the frame. The capability of the kidneys, intestines, pores and pores and skin, movement, and lungs is advanced via reflexology.

It will decorate the capability to manipulate the bladder and bowels. Reflexology relieves pain with the useful resource of stimulating the nerve terminals within the foot through the use of liberating endorphins (the body's herbal painkillers). It can lessen weariness and anxiety.

Reflexology allows alleviate the uncomfortable aspect consequences of many most cancers treatment options. As prolonged as you do not have a temperature, it gives treatment from colds and flu. It can help activate labor in past due pregnancies.

There are many blessings of reflexology. These benefits are physiological and intellectual. Reflexology can be a superb choice if you are searching for for possibility strategies to increase the mind's and frame's elegant efficacy! This is a confirmed and appealing approach for enhancing fitness without using chemical-based medicines and costly scientific treatments.

Chapter 4: How Does Reflexology Work?

Reflexology is a complementary remedy that treats congestion in exceptional "associated" quantities of the body with the useful resource of working on the foot. Reflexology is a slight remedy that restores and maintains the frame's natural balance.

Reflexology is incapable of curing any foremost or existence-threatening clinical situation and does now not promise to remedy, diagnose or prescribe; but, it is noticeably well-known amongst humans of all backgrounds as an opportunity recovery treatment.

Reflexology is suitable for each person. Many human beings use reflexology to lighten up the mind and body, and it's been established to be an powerful technique for:

Sleep issues.

Health disorders related to strain.

Backache.

Migraine.

Fertility problems.

Sleep issues.

Intestinal issues.

Hormonal imbalances.

Osteoarthritis.

Due to the occurrence of pressure in cutting-edge-day lifestyle, this moderate, calming treatment gives a way of pressure remedy that may be beneficial on a physical, intellectual and emotional diploma.

How Does Reflexology Function?

By using and stimulating pressure to the ft or fingers, reflexology can stimulate particular physiological and muscle sports activities.

The arms and feet are more sensitive than maximum people accept as true with. Reflexologists are knowledgeable to come across minute modifications in unique locations on the feet, and with the aid of way of manipulating the ones points, they could effect the right organ or body tool.

Studies have showed that reflexology improves bodily and emotional moves, boosts shallowness and self-self perception, and will boom motivation and popularity.

What Occurs During a Reflexology Treatment?

According to Chinese medicine, the sensory nerves of the frame's internal organs are located within the soles of the ft. During a reflexology remedy, the therapist applies guide pressure at the foot, operating on tremendous reflex points just like numerous frame zones.

Then, pressure is delivered to certain zones of the soles of the toes. Deposits and imbalances are recognized and removed to easy blockages and restore blood flow and strength.

Reflexology entails the usage of the fingers, hands, a timber stick, cream, and oils to prompt a reflex hobby in every other part of the frame. Reflexology, while nicely completed, induces a enjoy of nicely-being and relaxation at the same time as stimulating the frame to restore itself.

As virtually your shoes and socks might be removed, you ought to placed on unfastened, comfortable clothing that is not constricting.

Is reflexology secure for everyone?

Before starting reflexology, you need to visit your healthcare professional when you have a coronary coronary coronary heart illness, diabetes, epilepsy, excessive blood pressure, or kidney illness.

Women who are pregnant, menstruating, or bleeding internally or externally should now not undergo reflexology. Regular reflexology massages are permitted for a most of forty five mins. You must begin to see an improvement after one or treatments. Most people revel in a enjoy of nicely-being and rest.

Occasionally, people file experiencing nausea, tears, or lethargy following a reflexology treatment. According to therapists, this is part of the recuperation manner.

You ought to communicate any of those sensations in your reflexology therapist in order that she or he may be capable of alter your remedy plan consequently.

After eating, reflexology must be avoided for as a minimum one hour. You want to eat copious quantities of water following remedy as with different massage remedies.

Reflexology has currently increased in popularity as a manner of de-stressing and fun the thoughts and frame from the desires all people enjoy every day.

Chapter 5: Can Reflexology Assist With Back Pain?

Low lower returned pain extensively contributes to paintings absence, disability, and scientific fees. The predicted yearly direct fitness care charge of low decrease again pain inside the United Kingdom is form of £1.6 billion, making it one of the most steeply-priced clinical ailments within the united states of america of the united states.

It is thought that 60 and eighty percentage of the populace also can experience low again ache. Fifty percentage of low again ache episodes are anticipated to decrease inner four weeks; however, fifteen to twenty percent of sufferers experience pain after one year.

People have sought possibility varieties of treatment, inclusive of chiropractic or maybe reflexology, due to the truth traditional treatments do no longer thoroughly manage the issue.

Reflexology is an acupressure rub down method completed on the feet, arms, ears, and face.

Reflexology has existed in historical cultures for over 5,000 years on the idea that our our bodies are reflected in miniature in our ft and fingers. By stimulating those precise "reflex zones," we're able to beautify our not unusual health and properly-being.

Reflexology is not "recognized" with the resource of the usage of western treatment, and there can be restricted have a take a look at on it, however this has not averted it from gaining popularity.

The remedy makes use of the human body and does not claim to remedy ailments.

Reflexology is gaining popularity as a remedy for decrease once more ache due to the truth it's miles a non-invasive treatment that actively promotes relaxation to alleviate mild to extreme once more pain.

Back ache is one of the regions of reflexology that has had this type of top and a long way-attaining impact that more take a look at has been executed in this location than in every different. Forty participants with herniated discs had 3 reflexology durations consistent with week as part of a modest medical investigation; the effects recommended a reduction in pain (zero.75 on a scale of 4) in 25 of the 40 patients.

In 2008, pilot studies regarding 15 patients with low once more ache become completed (40 minutes of reflexology weekly for six weeks). Pain tiers reduced substantially in reflexology-dealt with patients compared to folks that received sham treatments.

Does this show the validity of reflexology?

Does this recommend that reflexology is powerful for everyone?

This remedy is especially effective for alleviating decrease back aches and pains for lots humans. As with all holistic remedies, whether or not herbal or clinical, a trial to decide its efficacy is continuously encouraged. Due to how reflexology is finished, the worst-case scenario is which you depart the consultation feeling extra relaxed.

Hand reflexology is captivating for the cause that it can be completed publicly and at any time. Also, while human beings don't forget reflexology, they evidently think about the toes, despite the fact that hand reflexology offers some blessings. For instance, it is able to be carried out while there may be no time or room to artwork fame up.

Hand reflexology is the proper natural therapy for self-assist because it is easy to investigate and follow.

Many humans employ a aggregate of self-help foot techniques, self-help hand techniques, and reflexology administered via a therapist or a few different man or woman. Consider and take a look at with reflexology for yet again pain; you've got were given no longer anything to lose.

Chapter 6: Reflexology And Bodywork

Most humans recognize that a whole frame or perhaps a smooth neck rub down feels incredible, however how many are aware of massage's proper benefits? (Also called Therapeutic massage and Medical massage.)

In the past, massages were appeared as a pricey and indulgence. Still, in recent years, increasingly more humans are getting aware of its benefits and receiving massages often.

More faculties are being built, and there are a growing shape of therapists. The medical community acknowledges that rub down can extensively reduce stress, purify the body via shifting lymphatic fluid and alleviate pain and pain.

Unfortunately, coverage businesses maintain to refuse coverage. We have to strongly endorse for this due to the fact maximum human beings can't have sufficient cash it frequently. The extra clinical data we are capable of provide, the extra the risk it is going to be covered in the future. Few people are acquainted with reflexology, now not just like the ones familiar with rub down remedy. WHAT is the definition of reflexology?

First, reflexology isn't always rub down, notwithstanding having some of the same benefits. Reflexology is the technological understanding based totally mostly on the premise that reflexes inside the fingers and ft correspond to all body additives. It is a specialised approach of exerting strain on those reflexes to get the desired effects. Its origins can be attributed to each Egyptian and Chinese civilizations.

Following her have a look at of Zone Therapy with Dr. Fitzgerald, Eunice Ingham created modern reflexology inside the United States at some level within the Nineteen Thirties. Based on her effects, she moreover created the legitimate copyrighted foot charts.

The key blessings of a reflexology treatment are assuaging strain and tension and enhancing glide (every blood and lymphatic).

Reflexology assists in normalizing physical functioning and achieving homeostasis.

According to docs, 75% of all illnesses are pressure-related. Due to the brilliant pressure-relieving outcomes of reflexology, many people achieve exceptional consequences, in particular when mixed with a healthy weight loss program and workout. Reflexology cannot exacerbate any state of affairs. Because simplest the fingers are executed, it's far a safe and effective method for enhancing health.

Typically, a affected character want to start with or three remedies every week for the number one many weeks. Then, treatment options is probably spaced out until the individual discovers what works wonderful. A collection of six treatments need to start to produce favorable consequences.

I strongly endorse that your reflexologist be licensed with the resource of way of a good school and which you keep away from going to a salon or spa to get your toes massaged.

Chapter 7: The Relationship Between Reflexology And Multiple Sclerosis

Over four hundred,000 Multiple Sclerosis sufferers within the United States, and almost hundred more are recognized weekly. It is anticipated that 2.Five million humans international be troubled with the aid of the situation.

Multiple sclerosis is a state of affairs that influences the myelin that surrounds the body's nerve fibers. The wrapping is a protective diploma that improves the nerves' capability.

It is recognized that after the myelin sheath is disrupted, important communique among the CNS and the relaxation of the body breaks down. This, in flip, causes the signs and symptoms and signs and symptoms and signs of more than one sclerosis, which we will communicate in a 2nd, as they could impair the eyes, muscles, coordination, ache sensations, and numbness, among one-of-a-kind troubles.

Multiple sclerosis (MS) has no recognised treatment, and no remedy has been evolved to address it. However, opportunity recovery methods have showed promise in dealing with MS symptoms and signs and symptoms and signs.

One definition of "sclerosis" is scarred tissue that has stiffened.

Scar tissue (moreover referred to as plaque or lesions) will interfere with the mind's functionality to engage with the relaxation of the concerned tool via the spinal wire. This can in the long run result in neurological signs and signs, collectively with physical and/or cognitive disability and neuropsychiatric contamination.

Multiple Sclerosis is a disease in which, for unexplained motives, the body's immune device has attacked the vital disturbing device. The charge and intensity with which signs rise up will vary, beginning from few signs and symptoms to sudden assaults with exceedingly symptomless relapses to a slow improvement from the begin over the years to a brief, regular raise or any combination of the previous.

Symptoms:

They declare that no MS patients have identical signs and symptoms. The sickness's improvement and symptomatology range from character to man or woman.

What are the results of interrupting the nerve transmissions exchanged every 2nd most of the brain and spine? In addition to trouble with movement, common organ functioning and cognitive competencies also may be impaired.

You can also moreover pay attention approximately exquisite signs and symptoms and signs and symptoms, which includes imbalance, vertigo, and dizziness. The perception of weird pores and pores and skin sensations, which incorporates itching, burning, tingling and/or tickling, numbness, and soreness within the limbs, mainly the extremities, is a common symptom of peripheral nerve damage. Also frequently mentioned is the feeling of "pins and needles," in particular in the toes, legs, fingers, and fingers.

Also, the abilities of the eyes (double or hazy imaginative and prescient) and the colon and bladder may be impaired.

Cognitive impairments, which include reminiscence troubles, the disability to treatment issues, or even interest span, are often observed via persistent fatigue. Other signs and symptoms and signs that allows you to arise masses less often but don't have any a whole lot an awful lot much less effect embody troubles with swallowing, speech impairments, being attentive to loss, and complications.

In addition to problems with motor coordination (tremors or even seizures), the illness-precipitated spasticity or spasms also can impact the inner organs. Urinary problems such as urgency (or hesitancy), frequency, and incontinence can be as a result of the ones spasms inside the bladder.

Some people will want rehabilitation to maintain or restore out of place important talents for every day residing. In addition, as a reflexologist, you may collaborate with distinct therapists, which consist of those that specialise in speech, physical, occupational, cognitive, and vocational remedies.

Despite the problem of treating a couple of sclerosis, many people have grew to emerge as to complementary and possibility remedy (CAM) to control their disease and alleviate their symptoms and symptoms and signs.

How does Reflexology help?

Therefore, the problem is: ought to reflexology be useful for Multiple Sclerosis sufferers? Can reflexology enhance the signs of multiple sclerosis? And, in that case, which of the numerous signs need to it help in alleviating?

Reflexologists can't address, diagnose or prescribe, as is not uncommon knowledge. Despite this, reflexology has emerge as a well-known supplemental remedy for more than one sclerosis. A massive quantity of research (supplied in my previous teleclass however too many to listing right right here) has already been finished on the control of:

bladder function.

pain.

numbness.

sleep troubles.

sleeplessness and sleep problems.

and further commonplace MS symptoms.

Approximately 50-60% of Multiple Sclerosis patients are presently believed to use complementary and possibility medicine (CAM). Meditation, Yoga, Tai Chi Chuan, Diets, Vitamin and Dietary Supplements, Naturopathy, Acupuncture, and Reflexology are well-known strategies.

It is well-known that reflexology can improve circulate, guide the immune device, and spark off many restoration energies. People with MS who get maintain of reflexology advise that treatment is beneficial for reducing all the signs and symptoms and signs and symptoms stated above, together with pain, bladder function, insomnia and sleep troubles, numbness, and strain.

We are aware that reflexology cannot replace traditional remedy. It enhances and assists the medical profession.

Multiple Sclerosis is a sickness with out a acknowledged treatment. Hence many physicians refer their MS patients to find out Complementary and Alternative Modalities.

Chapter 8: Reflexology To Assist With Labor Induction.

Reflexology can offer pressure and pain alleviation in a manner similar to that of massage. It is a supplementary treatment primarily based totally totally on the precept that precise frame elements correspond to particular factors on the toes. By utilising strain to targeted areas at the palms and feet, reflexology is generally used to relieve ache and anxiety.

Reflexology can play a characteristic in hard work induction. The therapist applies stress, stretches, and actions the complete foot in a few unspecified time within the future of the remedy. Reflexology have to not be painful, and the therapist have to art work in the affected person's consolation region.

Reflexology is a agency pressure applied to the foot that does not tickle. The treatment commences with a foot rub down. During the remedy, you could revel in numerous sensations for your feet and frame, which incorporates tingling or a hint pins-and-needles. Sensitivity differs among people and amongst remedies.

An hour-lengthy reflexology appointment have to encompass a consultation and an opportunity to discuss the treatment in a while. During pregnancy, maternity reflexology is adjusted to the dreams of the mom and infant.

Inducement of difficult artwork.

Most ladies move into hard art work really. When exertions is induced, it's miles initiated artificially. An induction might be prepared while a being pregnant exceeds 41 weeks and is deemed late.

Induction is generally administered among forty one and 40 weeks gestation to save you a pregnancy from persevering with beyond this aspect. Midwives and physicians employ specific techniques to spark off difficult work. To prompt difficult work, the midwife may additionally do a membrane sweep.

If this method fails, drug treatment is typically the following step. Chemical induction is executed within the hospital, in which every mom and baby should be constantly watched. Many ladies are adamant about keeping off a chemical induction of labor and looking for techniques to provoke their tough artwork. Reflexology for pregnant girls is a famous alternative.

The function of pregnancy reflexology in induction.

Reflexology has been carried out to spark off hard paintings or maybe lessen tough paintings pains. An growing quantity of midwives are mastering this particular foot rub down approach.

Maternity reflexology is applied in labor and shipping rooms throughout the globe to alleviate sufferers' ache and stimulate exertions. High-stress levels are not conducive to the onset of exertions, and there's not anything greater calming than a foot massage.

However, reflexology is even more beneficial because it objectives the right regions that could facilitate a quicker start. Thus, you need to go to a very skilled therapist. The therapist will start with a foot massage in advance than transferring to specific pressure spots at the ft and ankles. These particular elements can be identified to a reflexologist knowledgeable in maternity artwork.

If a contraction starts offevolved offevolved offevolved, the therapist will right away prevent utilizing strain. The factors can be touchy, and lots of girls have a sturdy pulling sensation in the foot and uterus. Also, the toddler may additionally moreover emerge as notably active.

Once the contraction ceases, they'll reapply beneath pressure. The therapist will avoid those reflexology spots until at the least the 41st week after your due date. You truly do not need to hurry the infant prematurely. It is high to get hold of common remedy for the duration of a being pregnant in vicinity of organized until delivery.

This not pleasant lessens anxiety however additionally, in my enjoy, has a extraordinary impact on newborns, as they seem calmer after shipping. In addition to balancing hormones, regulating the digestive tool, strengthening muscle and bone with advanced waft, and boosting the immune gadget, this is crucial at some stage in pregnancy, ordinary remedies might also repair hormonal stability, manage the digestive device, provide a lift to muscle and bone and raise the immune device.

It is important to understand that if the toddler isn't equipped to attain, now not some thing can change it! It can assist the frame in a laugh and making geared up for what is set to rise up.

Maintaining a pleasing mind-set within the days main as plenty as hard artwork is essential. If you start to have bad thoughts about childbirth, this can boom your stress tiers and postpone your tough work.

Try to count on your new infant with enthusiasm and pride. In typically, we want to awareness plenty much less on dashing the infants and extra on presenting emotional beneficial aid to the mom.

You can speak your anxieties with the therapist due to the fact they had been taught to understand the importance of extremely good questioning. They may be able to provide useful system, which consist of relaxation CDs or pleasant visualization sports.

By deciding on a complementary remedy like maternity reflexology to activate difficult art work, girls can revel in greater steady of their abilties to provide starting. Women who're aware of alternatives to scientific induction can repair a few control over their pregnancies in region of feeling at the mercy of scientific desire-makers.

Chapter 9: Prenatal Reflexology

Many midwives now use reflexology in their practices, demonstrating its efficacy. Maternity Reflexology can be used for preconception care and at some point of and after pregnancy. These lifestyles degrees offer specific traumatic conditions, and not unusual reflexology can help in retaining stability and well-being at the equal time as addressing associated ailments and illnesses.

Reflexology's capacity to stability the endocrine devicethe glands that create the body's hormonesis considered considered certainly one of its primary blessings (chemical messengers). Hormones are essential to fertility and pregnancy.

Pre-Conception.

For couples wishing to conceive, it is top-rated to cope with each companions to balance and loosen up them and located them in a kingdom this is top of the road for concept. In addition to healthful sperm and eggs, every companions require highbrow and emotional schooling, as being pregnant may be an emotional roller coaster. Creating each other individual is a specially critical project. Thus, it is prudent to be properly-organized.

The pair will need to have a look at their life-style in phrases of sleep, weight loss program, pressure levels, physical interest, smoking, ingesting, and many others. Due to its balancing results, reflexology has a tremendous popularity for assisting precept.

Pregnancy.

Not certainly physical however additionally psychologically, a pair undergoes extremely good adjustments inside the path of pregnancy. Things that formerly seemed to characteristic properly no longer seem to feature! Reflexology allows repair balance and harmony while you revel in the area has been flipped the alternative way up.

You may additionally enjoy abrupt constipation, bloating, acid reflux disorder ailment ailment, or burst into tears at the equal time as perusing baked beans in Sainsbury's. You can also have top notch abnormal aches and pains that emerge out of nowhere. You need to are looking for medical cope with primary being pregnant problems.

However, reflexology can assist inside the control of conditions which encompass:

Constipation.

Heartburn.

Symphysis pubis ache.

Backache.

Rib ache.

Morning nausea.

Leg cramps.

An prolonged blood stress.

Headaches.

fatigue and sleeplessness.

Mood swings.

Working with maternity reflexology has confirmed me the way it improves fitness and nicely-being whilst fostering a nurturing surroundings for the mom and the Incoming Soul (a lovable time period coined thru Susanne Enzer, maternity reflexologist).

I experience looking how energetic the unborn toddlers get while their mother is dealt with and noticing bottoms, heads, toes, and unique infant factors zipping around within the barriers of the little one bump!

Delivery.

After the due date and with the patron's and obstetrician's agreement, professional reflexology can help in inducing tough work. Many submit-term girls experiencing a trouble-loose pregnancy respond really to this, but in the long run, the infant makes a selection at the same time as to attain.

Not even clinical induction ensures fulfillment, and neither does this. Reflexologists may additionally moreover attend births to resource with pain management, relaxation, and emotional and psychological assist for the patron.

After Birth.

Your reflexologist can help the mom, father, and new child throughout postpartum. A weekly consultation can help the mother adjust to lifestyles as a ultra-modern mother, and he or she or he can breastfeed or hold the infant in the course of treatment.

Reflexology may additionally additionally promote lactation, alleviate breast discomfort or mastitis and assist the frame in returning to normal feature after childbirth. It also can assist new parents in adjusting emotionally and psychologically to parenthood.

Playing collectively together with your infant's ft and feet is a terrific way to bond together along with her or him. Finally, new child infants also can benefit from reflexology. Did you comprehend "This Little Piggy" is an edition of a top notch reflexology balancing technique?

You can play earlier than your toddler is going to mattress, during bathtub time, or even as you're winding them down after a feeding. Find a time this is conducive for each events. A reflexologist can educate you a few primary, calming movements to relieve your little one's troubles, which encompass colic, constipation, bad feeding, or sadness.

Chapter 10: Reflexology Is Significantly More Than A Foot Massage

So many people mistake reflexology with foot rub down by myself. If you're this form of humans, allow me to enlighten you. You are within the proper area in case you are seeking out facts that clarifies the severa misunderstandings round reflexology. The subsequent paragraphs will talk and offer an reason of the information of reflexology.

Reflexology is a manner in which a licensed therapist applies thumb and finger pressure to unique regions on the hands, ft, and even the ears. These locations are the body's reflex internet web sites. When those reflex internet net websites are massaged, pain remedy or an imbalance associated with a positive frame place is removed gently.

When your body's systems aren't functioning well, calcium, minerals, and uric acid deposits can also moreover moreover collect in the reflex net web sites, eventually impeding blood motion. A certified reflexologist can make use of rubdown techniques to remove those deposits and repair regular characteristic.

In addition, studies shows that 75% of ailments and problems are because of pressure. Resting and thrilling is the first step to preventing pressure-associated troubles. Here, reflexology comes into play. Concentrating at the reflex websites can assist the frame lighten up through regulating blood go together with the flow and soothing nerves, allowing the body to enjoy the whole blessings of reflexology.

Your palms and toes are constructed from many nerve endings that hyperlink to severa regions of your body. After locating and massaging the superb places of your ft and hands, you may stimulate the affected areas of your body.

Although reflexology also can be done at the arms, maximum reflexologists prefer to massage the feet because of the truth that they're large and further handy. This is why many people mistake reflexology for a easy foot massage.

Hand reflexology is appropriate for individuals who dislike massaging or studying their ft and those who be troubled by way of hand ailments like arthritis or carpal tunnel syndrome.

Hand reflexology may be finished everywhere with out feeling traumatic, in contrast to foot reflexology. However, abuse of the palms may additionally motive them to become plenty less sensitive, which could on occasion lessen the efficacy of this form of reflexology.

Increasing numbers of people now flip to alternative treatments like reflexology, likely as it promises minimal horrific results. It also can take a few instructions of reflexology before you enjoy its effects, however you may quick realize that it's miles honestly useful and effective.

Reflexology images and charts are to be had to examine wherein and to which reflex points to apply pressure. Attending a reflexology software or path is exceedingly advocated in case you choice an entire training in reflexology.

You can exercise the strategies you studies for yourself. Still, reflexology is extra effective while achieved via any other individual, permitting you to lighten up greater and improving the body's recovery strength.

A wealth of assets are to be had to help you analyze the precise reflexology elements and stress, or you could attend nighttime training to collect the know-how you can want for your home treatments or private instructions.

If you endorse to use your information and training professionally, you can start acting reflexology in your circle of relatives. This will serve functions: introducing them to the advantages of reflexology and allowing you to benefit enjoy and remarks. Remember that reflexology is only effective whilst completed efficaciously. Therefore, do not try to exercise it with out the preferred studies and training.

Long misunderstood, reflexology is now becoming identified as more than quality a foot massage. There is a scientific foundation for the remedy, and its efficacy has been drastically verified.

Chapter 11: Hands Reflexology As A Healing Art

Reflexology is a not unusual technique that includes using pressure to particular strain points. These zones correspond to the pressure factors on the human body. This method applies to every the fingers and feet. Reflexology on the hands dates again to historical Egypt.

Today, there are even extra advantages at hand reflexology. Daily use of game consoles, laptops, and special handheld digital gadgets consequences in immoderate hand use. Hand reflexology is beneficial for overworked palms because it relaxes the palms and the complete body.

Hand reflexology is crucial if you are searching out a manner to disrupt the stress cycles for your frame. As pressure sensors are stimulated with the useful resource of hand reflexology, corresponding body areas become comfortable. As this rest travels via the nerve device, it spreads within the course of the frame.

As the body is de-careworn and cushty, restoration can start, and fitness may moreover decorate. According to medical research, meditation and reflexology positively have an effect on the thoughts and coronary heart.

Hand reflexology isn't always as famous as foot reflexology, however every strategies carry out further. Because palms are more efficaciously to be had and we are familiar with working with them, many people discover them plenty less tough to control.

Anyone can have a look at hand reflexology. It is a number one technique that includes mixing motion, stress, and stretches to break the built pressure patterns. As you exercise hand reflexology, keep away from overworking your palms; when you have any ache or ache after a reflexology session, you should go away your palms to relaxation for a few days.

You may additionally even hold close the strategies of hand reflexology and lease them your self. These strategies are nice if you want a few moments to loosen up or sense stressful.

Finding a reputable source of records and learning the processes is simple. Many belongings provide step-thru-step commands for treatments and maps indicating which quantities of your hands connect to specific frame zones.

Many human beings enjoy making use of pressure with massage implements. There are inexperienced timber devices for exciting stress points that may be rolled among the hands.

Kevin Kunz, a reflexologist from the United Kingdom, claims his favored tool for hand reflexology is a gold ball. "Grasp the palms collectively on the equal time as protective a golfing ball many of the palms and roll the ball throughout the palm below the thumb," he shows.

Chapter 12: The Reflexology Method For Sciatica Relief

You may additionally enjoy it's miles a waste of time to analyze this remedy for sciatica remedy because of the fact it's far unconventional. If you have not professional foot reflexology, you could marvel how the use of stress to nice areas on the bottoms of your toes or arms may additionally moreover alleviate sciatica. Allow me to elaborate in advance than you brush aside this non-surgical alternative.

First and essential, what is reflexology, and the manner can it aid returned or exceptional body imbalances?

Reflexology is the software of thumb, finger, and hand techniques or (in the east) a tool based totally totally on a device of zones symbolizing the frame at the feet and palms with the resource of a therapist (or oneself).

The principle is based on the belief that electricity channels flow right faraway from the soles of the toes or the hands to the organs. Another concept is that nerves pass from the fingers or soles of the ft to remarkable frame regions.

Allow me to apply the preceding in your lower again or sciatica pain. Imagine that a muscular inflammation motives your sciatica. How can one benefit consolation from sciatica? Reflexology has been validated to set off relaxation, relieve pain, decorate blood stream, and assist.

This scenario is using strain to the sciatic nerve. A foot replicate should enhance blood circulate. When in assessment with rubdown, reflexology offers the same advantages. Both treatments enhance blood go together with the float to the affected muscle, this is beneficial. I strongly propose you provide reflexology a strive!

What is worried in a foot reflexology session? The intention is to facilitate get proper of access to to the toes for the reflexologist. Typically, the affected person sleeps on a massage bed or recliner-style chair. Typically, the therapist will use massage oil or cream to facilitate the smooth passage of pressure elements.

Once both the therapist and consumer are organized, the consultation will start. Most schooling could in all likelihood run among 20 and 50 mins. The therapist threatens via the use of utilising stress on the organ-imparting websites. The therapist could observe the client's pain place and skin discoloration.

The patron can also moreover additionally enjoy a sensation much like crystals being overwhelmed. When administering reflexology, I request that the patron rest even as I work at the toes. Also, it's far essential to have at least one eight-ounce glass of water right now after the exercise. Why drink water?

Chapter 13: Reflexology For Muscle And Joint Pain

Reflexology is using pressure with the thumb and fingers to responsive spots at the ft and hands to stimulate bodily skills. It has been examined that this stimulation induces physiological modifications inside the frame and want to not be burdened with rubdown. Massage targets the underlying area being impacted, while, in reflexology, the vicinity being labored on creates adjustments in a super body place.

For a long term, reflexology has been stated to have preventative and restoration advantages at the frame. It has presently won recognition as a remedy for muscle and joint ache and persistent ache. The frame want to be handled as a whole. When treating ache; reflexology effectively treats the frame and assists in preventing future ailments.

Reflexology is an splendid possibility remedy for foot pain because it addresses the hassle's essential purpose. Reflexology has been examined to be in particular effective in treating foot ache. Various forms of reflexology have alleviated specific situations, which includes bunions, swollen ft, and joint disjunction.

Since it's miles been examined that over seventy-five percentage of illnesses are stress-related or may be cured via using casting off the stressor, reflexology has gained legitimacy.

According to the thoughts of reflexology, many illnesses are because of an accumulation of chemicals mainly frame factors, collectively with the palms and feet. Stimulating the ones areas can destroy down the accumulation and alleviate the symptoms and signs.

Calcium and uric acid are minerals appeared to generate buildups and impair the perfect operation of the frame, which includes blood go along with the glide and organs. This might also additionally have negative effects at the joints, resulting in pain. Allowing the ones mineral deposits to be discharged can reduce the strain on the joints causing discomfort.

Each foot contains greater than seven thousand nerve endings related to the thoughts. This reality begins to provide reflexology the value it merits.

Reflexology has been verified to alleviate the signs of arthritis in a trial regarding about one thousand people. Twenty-six bones make up the hand. All those bones need to act in stay general performance to advantage suitable functioning of the hand and wrist. The manipulation of these bones can notably lessen arthritic ache.

Reflexology is started out to be included with the aid of manner of way of increasingly fitness suggestions.

Chapter 14: How To Detoxify Your System Using Reflexology

Did you apprehend that reflexology can help with body detoxification? Reflexology is primarily based on the premise that reflex factors or zones at the foot correspond to inner frame points, organs, and systems. The practitioner can address areas of illness, imbalance, or weakness thru manipulating these zones and elements.

Since Egyptian times, reflexology has been documented, and Eunice Ingham documented the exercise within the early 1900s. Ingham, a physiotherapist, felt that the frame consisted of many interconnected zones.

She believed these might be accessed and dealt with extra without issue in particular physical regions, collectively with the foot. This paintings led to the development of reflexology as it is practiced nowadays.

During a reflexology session, the client sits or reclines on a couch whilst the practitioner follows a chain of manipulations round each foot, encompassing all reflex elements and zones. During remedy, the practitioner will request patron comments on any areas of discomfort or ache. The practitioner can "art work" the affected region to relieve the trouble.

Reflexology is an amazing diagnostic method for the reason that it is able to find out troubles in the body, even in its earliest ranges. The practitioner can then address them earlier than extra, greater intense problems get up. Reflexology practitioners typically make use of powders including calendula or talcum to facilitate the remedy.

During a detox eating regimen ordinary, your inner organs and systems will in all likelihood feature greater hard or otherwise than they typically ought to. Reflexology can useful resource the body's detoxification way thru 'balancing' organs together with the kidneys and liver and allowing the intestines to perform their cleansing with out exerting undue stress.

Reflexology can also screen what your body desires or what it's miles experiencing. If you obtain reflexology treatments on the identical time as detoxifying your frame, you will locate that the maximum common "sensitive elements" are those of the running-tough bladder, kidney, and digestive structures. The practitioner will art work on those places to beautify their situation for further cleansing.

Also, reflexology treatments will screen any viable imbalance, allowing the practitioner to take precautionary measures. Reflexology remedies are still beneficial as a preventative degree and a way to unwind even in case you are in excellent fitness or if a detox has left your body genuinely balanced.

There are a few number one reflex spots that may be worked on every day to promote serenity and health:

The "awesome eliminator," placed the various thumb and forefinger, can be applied to release anxiety and stress. Using your left thumb and arms, lightly compress this fleshy place on your proper hand.

As it can be painful, you ought to observe strain cautiously, mainly when you have a headache or are tense—over and over applying and freeing strain until the tension or headache subsides. When you revel in prepared, transfer arms and release tension inside the precise hand.

The 'center factor' within the palm of your hand corresponds to the 'center component' on your sun plexus (chest location) and the 'center aspect' for your foot; even though, your hand is the nice to attain.

Place your left thumb in the center of your right palm and use your left arms to guide the weight of your proper hand. Slowly increase the thumb upwards closer to the hands and prevent while the lowest of the knuckles is reachedslightly off-center from the palm to the arms. Again, cautiously exercise strain and keep it till it decreases. Repeat for the opposite hand, and you could revel in the anxiety expend.

You can control the region elements for your face via manner of putting each thumbs proper internal the attention socket in the route of the brow bone. Place your elbows on a desk or table and decrease your head onto your thumbs. Maintain the strain, then release it. Again, this may sense sore, particularly in case you try to alleviate a headache.

There are severa tactics to detoxify your frame, and complementary recuperation procedures consisting of reflexology are a top notch technique to casting off pollution from your device. When you start reading the way to cleanse your frame, indulge yourself and attempt a modern-day remedy each couple of weeksthe strive might be properly in reality worth it.

Chapter 15: Reflexology For Rejuvenation

Foot reflexology is a natural method of rejuvenation and healing, and you may be astonished with the resource of its efficacy. Learn how this foot rub down can benefit you whilst no longer having medicine. You will probably want first of all the aid of learning the origins of reflexology and the manner it came into exercise.

Reflexology originated in Middle Eastern international locations like China and Egypt. The toes have around 7,000 nerve endings, which may be inspired with foot rub down. Those who spend loads of time on their toes can benefit substantially from reflexology as a recovery useful useful aid. So, what advantages are you capable of anticipate from this shape of remedy?

You would possibly likely already count on reflexology is pretty calming however also can offer you with different fitness advantages. It now not fine revitalizes you and improves your blood motion, however it could furthermore assist you remove built-up stress on your frame. It accomplishes this through relieving muscle anxiety and enhancing the immune system. Many studies have tested that it may additionally growth hobby.

There may not be instant outcomes after your first reflexology consultation, but you can clearly enjoy more cushty. Typically, it takes a couple of training in advance than you begin to be aware the real advantages of rejuvenation on your complete body. Don't, therefore, stop after the primary consultation. Instead, make sure which you touch your reflexologist frequently to get the ones advantages.

Many human beings see a reflexologist to revitalize and revive themselves to have extra power inside the direction in their day by day sports activities sports. You may additionally enjoy an boom in strength after a reflexology consultation. This may be beneficial.

If you expect hard situations, along with checks, a brand new project, or a float, do no longer wait until you are careworn to put together. Schedule an appointment along side your reflexologist and get a burst of strength in advance to get you thru each day traumatic conditions.

Almost truly anyone will discover this a calming experience that notably contributes to their normal fitness. Not first-rate also can it help you decorate the stability of your fitness, but it is able to additionally get rid of each day stressors. Not to say the fact that your training offer you with a exceptional deal-preferred by myself time.

Don't be concerned approximately the actual consultation. Some people worry that the Reflexology consultation may be daunting, mainly within the event that they've ticklish or sensitive feet. Your reflexologist may be capable of regulate the amount of strain they look at based totally truely at the degree of sensitivity to your ft.

Chapter 16: Reflexology And Seniors

Reflexology and dealing with the elderly sound like a in form made in heaven. Alternatives to drugs are typically more secure and function fewer trouble results. Thus, they're usually of interest.

Reflexology is undeniably powerful, as evidenced as an extended way lower lower back as historic instances. People generally appear revitalized after a reflexology consultation; inside the event that they do not, their our bodies require extra rest. In addition to nursing houses accepting reflexology as an powerful more and opportunity treatment, reflexology has additionally located an area in eldercare and hospice.

Reflexology performed thru a properly-professional reflexologist can make contributions appreciably to stepped forward fitness or a faster restoration.

Here are some reasons reflexology is so essential in hospices and nursing homes:

Reflexology alleviates pain, honestly making someone enjoy first-class and snug. It may additionally furthermore reduce the want for painkillers with ability negative consequences, but simplest a medical professional can decide this.

It can assist a person sense revitalized with reduced stiffness, allowing them to engage in every day sports with more ease and luxury.

Reflexology improves the drift of blood. Increased move expedites the recuperation way. It can also decorate lymph, neuron, and muscle characteristic.

The customer can get and experience the blessings at the same time as seated or lying down; there can be no want to roll over or get rid of clothing.

Reflexology improves body consciousness and stimulates the neurological device. Better nerve feature can beneficial useful resource keep quicker reflexes, allowing one to govern ordinary sports better.

Furthermore, reflexology is a consistent and empathetic contact that is not overly invasive.

Even whilst residing in centers which include nursing homes, a wonderful a part of the population, the elderly, can experience by myself and lonely. The touch they get hold of in establishments is typically realistic and often mechanical, making reflexology a in particular valued revel in due to its attentive and non-invasive attributes.

There are some issues to maintain in mind at the same time as operating with the elderly:

Always are looking for advice from a systematic practitioner earlier than starting to paintings with someone with fitness worries, because the elderly commonly have a propensity to be afflicted by using more ailments and characteristic more complications. This is significantly much less complicated to perform even as the affected individual is in a nursing home or hospice, in which medical experts are on employees.

Use less stress on the identical time as starting to artwork with elderly customers, as their organ systems are possibly to be slow due to their superior age. There isn't any need to delve too deeply or too quick, particularly earlier than identifying the affected person's tolerance for reflexology and possibly in no way if running in a hospice putting.

Reduce the period of the consultation; there may be no need to exhaust the frame. The restoration advantages are but present; you may not exceed their goals or desires with a shorter consultation.

Chapter 17: How Reflexology Can Improve Your Health

The present day-day life-style entails a number of stress and worry. There are many reasons of tension and pressure, which incorporates stress, competitiveness, office and circle of relatives control, and so on. In such situations, it's far critical to rest and renew the frame. Reflexology is a super way to unwind the frame.

Do each day aches and pains drain your power? In this situation, you could discover the numerous techniques beneficial. Reflexology is a charming form of complementary treatment. Reflexology specializes inside the ears, fingers, and toes as particular zones. Most of the time, it takes area on the foot due to the truth there are loads more areas to deal with.

If you have were given were given formerly tried reflexology to your palms with out achievement, I endorse you to attempt it all over again for your toes. They are associated with greater emotions, and you'll find that you may revel in greater via this technique than together in conjunction with your arms or ears. The appropriate amount of pressure performed to the vicinity can also affect the outcomes.

People occasionally discover that combining reflexology with effective important oils yields even higher benefits. Ensure that the crucial oils you operate correspond to the popular results of the reflexology. There is massive statistics about this available on-line and in print.

Have you obtained a foot rub down and felt proper away happier? Perhaps it revitalized you and gave you more strength than you've got got had in a totally long term. These are common benefits of reflexology from which you can benefit. If the techniques are completed by way of someone who has researched the diverse places on the body, unique illnesses may be alleviated.

Do you experience chronic headaches?

Perhaps you have tried many remedies without achievement. Reflexology techniques may additionally moreover provide you with longed-for independence from them. This is because of the relationship amongst strain spots at the body and lots of receptors in the frame and mind.

It is fascinating to have a have a look at a reflexology chart because it depicts the regions of the toes that correspond to different body sections. You can find out the areas from which you need to derive blessings. If you're interested in experimenting with reflexology at home, home check courses teach you the basics.

Even even though many claims they have by no means skilled such relief earlier than reflexology, the scientific global remains quite suspicious of it. Many professionals experience it is largely a precept of mind over recollect; if you want reflexology to be powerful, you can obtain the favored effects.

Since the scientific community does not drastically apprehend reflexology, there are few licensing necessities. Nonetheless, you may look at that an increasing number of humans are training reflexology. Take the time to inquire approximately their credentials. You need someone who has completed the favored guides to manage it.

Reflexology is an top notch treatment for treating illnesses, fun the body, and serving as a preventative remedy. It is an exceptional approach to resource the body's restoration method. Everyone can advantage from reflexology, from new infant toddlers to humans of their very last days.

Listening to our our our bodies is the maximum vital day by day project all and sundry must conduct, however we fail to advantage this. We have to come to be aware about what pressure seems like and what troubles our our our our bodies are experiencing. We want to begin to pay attention to our our our bodies and sense what pressure is doing to them. How often do you have got slight lower lower back ache and blunder it for strain?

Small aches and pains want to be recommended to the scientific clinical doctor right now. You need to recognize that those seemingly risk free symptoms and signs and symptoms ought to result in severe outcomes. Consult a medical doctor right now if you are experiencing a scenario or pain.

Another alternative is reflexology. One might have reflexology treatment for the organ that is generating issues. There are a few factors to keep in mind whilst receiving reflexology for a specific trouble.

Without schooling, you need to no longer workout reflexology for your private. It is wonderful to are looking for out a qualified therapist. If the situation persists, you need to go to a clinical doctor without delay and stop reflexology.

Sometimes you aren't really cured of a effective contamination or illness however feel you've got recovered. You forestall your remedy and indulge. In such events, reflexology is normally recommended to save you relapse. Reflexology is every preventative and healing.

Reflexology is so stunning that it may deal with troubles related to all five senses: sight, smell, sound, touch, and taste. It can free someone from their addictions, erase and alleviate the ache of arthritis and cancer, get to the bottom of the hassle and assist it, put off worry and guilt, promote speedy restoration and yield the blessings of a extra information of oneself.

Many advantages are related to reflexology remedies, but what is reflexology, and why need to we do not forget utilizing it?

Living in the present day-day global has many boundaries, in conjunction with very last physical in form and healthy. As a culture, we're often overworked, exhausted, and pressured and do now not care for ourselves. However, there are techniques to be had to triumph over every of those problems.

Reflexology is a technology as it includes massaging precise reflexes or stress factors inside the ft, hands, and ears. This will correspond to amazing body sections.

As an example, a hand reaction might also additionally relieve the lower back muscle businesses or knee pain. Reflexology is a whole remedy, which means that it is a natural treatment. It is becoming increasingly apparent that herbal healing, in preference to the use of risky drug treatments, is the critical aspect to maintaining humans wholesome.

Reflexology is powerful as it stimulates reflex spots in the arms, toes, and ears. These regions are interconnected with all frame components, which incorporates muscle groups, tissues, and organs.

The corresponding physical element is harmonized and purified thru exerting gentle pressure on superb locations. Reflexology remedies are powerful due to the fact they lighten up the frame, alleviate tension and promote self-restoration with the aid of the use of using releasing congestion in the affected regions.

After their first reflexology treatment, most humans will probably believe they have visited a spa in choice to acquired remedy. Typically, a visit starts offevolved with a consultation with a professional reflexologist.

Depending on wherein remedy need to begin, the affected person may be counseled to lie down or live seated. The reflexologist will then rub down the fingers and toes, applying mild stress to the areas much like the sick body. Patients also can require a couple of treatments to fulfill their frame's requirements.

The advantages of reflexology are many. They relieve ache and tension, enhance blood go with the flow, gain concord, and get rid of pollutants. Here are some information on how reflexology assists with some of our maximum vital fitness troubles.

Stress can seem in loads of methods within the body, with tension headaches, migraines, constipation, and pimples frequently the maximum glaring. Reflexology can assist with the resource of way of loosening strain's grip on the frame and assuaging its symptoms and signs.

Reflexology additionally offers natural and effective ache remedy. Pain is mostly a caution signal sent with the beneficial aid of the body even as some factor is inaccurate. All too often, ache is a issue impact of physical recovery, whether or now not or now not by way of the usage of manner of medicinal capsules or surgical treatment. Reflexology can alleviate this ache by means of manner of guiding the frame to restore itself via the release of endorphins.

Reflexology has been installation to be one of the handiest possibility remedies for keeping physical health. Asthma, bronchitis, premenstrual syndrome and one-of-a-kind fitness conditions have furthermore established extensive treatment with reflexology remedies. However, patients want not wait till they're unwell to are in search of a expert reflexologist.

As with extraordinary alternative medicinal drug, you should decide whether reflexology can offer your selected advantages. Why now not deliver it a shot when you have been laid low with many troubles for some time? You may furthermore discover that it's far a natural and less expensive manner to sense your greatest all over again.

Chapter 18: The Relaxing Path To Health And Wellness Through Reflexology

Traditional rubdown techniques for muscle anxiety release and rest are widely known. Many people moreover know that making use of strain to particular locations at the palms can alleviate a headache and that massaging particular places on the ankles can set off hard paintings in a pregnant girl.

However, did you recognize that those are just a few secrets and techniques of the therapeutic method referred to as reflexology?

Although reflexology is normally called "foot massage," it's far a whole lot greater. Reflexology is a natural recovery method regarding the software program of pressure to nice spots on the foot that correspond to frame systems and organs.

According to the concept, underlying reflexology, "reflex" zones on the ft and fingers correlate to specific organs, glands, and special body components. For example:

The suggestions of the toes mirror the pinnacle.

The torso and coronary coronary heart are placed in the direction of the ball of the foot.

The pancreas, liver, and kidney are placed in the foot's arch.

The low back and intestines are positioned inside the course of the heel.

So, what's reflexology? Reflexology is a hand and foot rubdown that gives basic health blessings. Each frame's organs and systems correspond to particular spots on the ft and arms, which form the concept of reflexology. By the use of pressure to those regions, a practitioner can restore a proper stability to the frame. In western reflexology, the practitioner clearly uses her hands.

In the japanese shape of reflexology, system are applied further to the hands. Regardless of the fashion, a reflexologist uses charts highlighting specific areas that might help restore fitness issues or keep the frame's balance.

Although reflexology is an established technique that could assist in treating many minor and chronic health conditions, it is not a remedy. Reflexology have to complement medical remedy plans, not update them, for human beings with excellent health issues.

Reflexology is a supplementary remedy that treats a person holistically on a physical, emotional, highbrow, and spiritual diploma. It is a herbal, non-invasive therapy that encourages the frame's self-restoration houses.

Reflexology can be used to address a large type of illnesses, which include:

Allergies.

Migraines and headaches.

Back troubles.

Digestive issues.

Rheumatism.

PMT.

Fertility loss.

Indications of pregnancy.

Depression.

MS.

ME.

Melanoma.

Strain.

Stress.

Every day, many humans artwork while status and moving round on their ft. By together with reflexology treatments into your fitness and health regimen, you may also be capable of lessen the occurrence of numerous ailments.

Through reflexology, we are capable of transmit unique recuperation energies or restoration radiation into the strength fields of some different person to motive them to revel in better right away. In addition to relieving complications, backaches, or even heart pain, reflexology offers the recipient extra more youthful electricity and an immediate feel of properly-being.

Pain is the frame's manner of handing over a warning sign thru reflexes on the same time as some element is inaccurate. Simply positioned, exercise pressure or massage it everywhere you sense even the slightest ache to your frame. There can be a blockage or disease in a selected body area.

Expectations During Reflexology Treatment

Most reflexology durations take amongst 30 and 60 minutes. The consumer relaxes on a reclined chair with their ft and palms indoors smooth attain of the therapist. The reflexologist will control the feet and/or palms with the useful resource of using strain, stretching and movement.

Like big massage remedy, the reflexologist will reply on your caution symptoms and signs and symptoms regarding pressure and luxury. However, in evaluation to massage, reflexology is a dry approach that does not embody the use of creams or oils. Ensure that your goals are communicated at some stage in the consultation.

Enjoy the treatment in silence or request a customized evaluation of strain triggers and education in enforcing self-reflexology practices at domestic to hold the advantages following treatment.

Reflexology may be the last "Great Escape" in case you be concerned by way of manner of a sure situation or in case you really want an extraordinary foot rub down that leaves you with a experience of properly-being.

Chapter 19: Faq's On Reflexology

What is reflexology?

Reflexology stretches lower lower back at the least 5,000 years to ancient Egyptian and Oriental cultures. Because specific factors and goal regions manual practitioners of every strategies, some check it to acupuncture.

However, acupuncture consists of the software program of small needles to the entire body, at the same time as reflexology is needle-unfastened and makes a speciality of the toes. Also, reflexology can be done at the hands and ears.

Reflexology perspectives the ft as miniature representations of the human body, with each organ, gland, and body detail having a matching reflex area or point within the foot. Reflexology expedites the comfort of the associated physical problem via focusing on a specific vicinity or aspect.

A reflexologist can useful resource the recovery of certain ailments via walking on exquisite regions of the toes; but, it is most dependable to balance the complete frame via jogging on all areas.

As an example of approaches reflexology can assist with healing or in fact alleviate ache and suffering, proper right right here are some examples: Menstrual cramps are not unusual. These are the elements of the foot that a reflexologist might also moreover popularity on: The ankle, the inner foot's most function, and the Heel.

The location of the frame that corresponds to the ones places at the foot: System of duplicate

Back, shoulder, and neck pain.

Reflexologists may also additionally consciousness on the following elements of the foot: The nook of the Foot's Insole.

The region of the body that corresponds to those places on the feet is: Spine.

Constipation and distinctive gastrointestinal problems A reflexologist can also give attention to the following components of the foot: The Arch's indoors.

The essential and minor intestines are the physical parts that correlate to the ones foot locations. Relaxation may be finished by means of reflexology because it helps the body alter and balance itself.

Additionally, reflexology creates a enjoy of calm that seems to wrap across the frame and permits the body and thoughts to release electricity go with the flow in addition to the proper effects that have been found, which includes good deal in migraines, constipation, cold/flu signs and signs, again/neck ache.

As a give up give up end result, you may have extra power, stamina, intellectual readability, and a more balanced emotional state. Even individuals tormented by prolonged-time period ailments like hypersensitive reactions, drug dependence, and weight reduction issues say they have got seen giant development in their situations.

Is Reflexology a form of medicine? No. Reflexology is neither a scientific method nor a foot rub down. Instead, reflexology is a terrific herbal recovery method. It is a technological know-how that involves test, sound approach, and practiced capabilities and an art work that takes passion and perseverance.

Is Reflexology painful? Rarely does a consumer declare discomfort in some unspecified time in the future of a reflexology consultation. Each foot includes twenty-six bones, fifty-six ligaments, thirty-8 muscle organizations, and 7 thousand neurons; consequently, many territories are stimulated at some point of a session.

During a reflexology session, emotions are sensed within the ft, no longer within the corresponding organs, glands, or different regions. Nonetheless, it is conventional for a client to experience soreness in one-of-a-kind regions of his or her body 1-2 days after a session.

During a session, pollutants are expelled from the ft, and it takes time for the body's natural elimination mechanism to smooth them out. It is counseled that the patron and therapist have an open dialogue to maximize the consumer's consultation.

Who presently makes use of Reflexology? Reflexology is simple to take a look at but pretty effective. Surgeons and different scientific specialists, chiropractors, podiatrists, dentists, nurses, midwives, physical therapists, occupational therapists, and rub down therapists lease it as a complementary modality.

Imagine the following situation to demonstrate the manner it is probably carried out at the issue of scientific practices: A pregnant girl is presently in difficult paintings. Although a number of her sufferings are treatable with modern-day pills, she maintains to have pain and pain in her decrease again and neck.

Reflexology is finished on the internal edges of her feet to help ease her neck and lower lower back ache; this is a fairly non-invasive remedy for an indoors sickness. There are not any needles, and not anything other than her feet should be uncovered.

In lots much less than an hour, she regains her composure, and her neck and decrease once more soreness subsides, permitting her to interest at the marvel of difficult art work! In addition, many thrilling non-experts pick to examine reflexology to alleviate pressure in their daily lives or the lives in their loved ones.

Is Reflexology a secure exercising? Reflexology is safe for all of us. This protected youngsters and the elderly. Frequent classes can advantage specific persistent illnesses, collectively with diabetes, maximum cancers, addictions, terminal contamination, and weight issues.

Chapter 20: The History Of Reflexology

Reflexology, an possibility medicinal approach, includes the stimulation of particular regions of the palms, ft, or ears, which promotes recovery in corresponding regions of the frame.

Despite being exceedingly modern, reflexology has roots dating lower returned millennia and has a rich and storied records that spans more than one cultures.

The complexity of reflexology's origins is intertwined with the earliest of civilizations, as evidenced by hieroglyphics depicting foot massages in ancient Egyptian tombs relationship again to 2330 BCE.

In historical China and India, reflexology become employed to promote relaxation and alleviate ache.

This recovery exercise have become known as "zoku shin do" or "foot reading" in traditional Chinese treatment.

Practitioners could meticulously scrutinize the ft to understand any physical imbalances, after which they might examine stress to unique elements to sell recovery.

Reflexology furthermore determined an area in Ayurvedic medication, one of the international's oldest holistic recuperation structures, where it turn out to be implemented to promote everyday well-being.

The nineteenth and 20th centuries noticed the emergence of reflexology within the West manner to pioneers together with William Fitzgerald and Eunice Ingham.

A scientific health practitioner of ear, nostril, and throat named Fitzgerald advanced the location treatment principle, which postulated that the human body ought to in all likelihood be divided into 10 vertical zones, every of which corresponded to a one in every of a kind hassle of the frame.

By applying pressure to unique factors in every quarter, Fitzgerald believed he need to alleviate pain and promote recuperation.

Ingham, a physiotherapist, similarly superior Fitzgerald's paintings through the use of focusing on the feet as the number one area for reflexology.

Today, reflexology is a sought-after complementary treatment practiced international, which promotes relaxation, reduces strain, alleviates pain, and enhances ordinary health and well-being.

Reflexologists operate in various settings, which include spas, well-being centers, and hospitals, and may be certified with the useful resource of professional corporations similar to the Reflexology Association of America or the International Institute of Reflexology.

Reflexology stays a valuable addition to conventional clinical cures for many human beings, regardless of the reality that it's far yet to be clinically tested as a way to deal with any unique ailment or contamination.

In quit, the complexity and diversity of reflexology's origins and development have set up it as a long lasting recovery exercise.

From historical Egypt to fashionable-day America, reflexology has been carried out to sell recuperation and enhance standard properly-being.

Its reputation and effectiveness as a complementary treatment are simple, no matter the mystery that also surrounds how reflexology works.

THE PRINCIPLES OF REFLEXOLOGY

Reflexology is a fascinating possibility remedy technique that includes making use of strain to specific points on the feet, fingers, and ears.

The idea is rooted within the perception that those elements correspond to severa organs and systems in the frame.

By using strain to the ones factors, reflexologists posit that they can stimulate the frame's herbal recuperation strategies, promoting not unusual fitness and properly-being.

A cornerstone principle of reflexology is the belief that the frame is a holistic machine with all factors interconnected and interdependent.

Consequently, the disorder of one detail can ripple and have an impact on different elements of the body as well.

By correcting abnormalities and obstructions within the movement of power, or qi, reflexology desires to reestablish the frame's equilibrium and harmony.

This will assist the frame get better itself extra short and efficaciously.

Moreover, reflexologists recall that absolutely everyone is unique, with their very personal set of health desires and stressful conditions, and consequently, require individualized treatment.

To layout a personalized remedy plan, reflexologists take a holistic technique, considering absolutely everyone's bodily, emotional, and spiritual health.

This tailored technique differs from a device that works for all of us.

Additionally, reflexology is a complementary treatment to specific clinical treatments, making it a popular desire to alleviate ache, lessen strain and tension, enhance flow into, and sell rest.

Reflexology's non-invasive nature moreover makes it a secure and gentle remedy for people of every age.

In summary, the thoughts of reflexology underscore the interconnectedness of the body, emphasizing the significance of restoring balance and concord to sell regular health and nicely-being.

By targeted on imbalances and blockages within the drift of energy, reflexology dreams to stimulate the body's natural restoration techniques and encourage green and effective recovery.

With its recognition on individualized remedy and herbal recuperation, reflexology is a moderate and effective remedy for promoting gold general fitness.

THE BENEFITS OF REFLEXOLOGY

Reflexology, a complementary treatment that applies strain to particular elements at the feet, hands, or ears, is gaining reputation due to its severa and wide-ranging blessings for giant health and nicely-being.

Reflexology is a technique that makes use of stress on the foot to promote the healing mechanisms of the frame and relieve some of symptoms and illnesses, along side migraines, cramping sooner or later of menstruation, and gastric issues.

By enhancing flow into, lowering inflammation, and stimulating the release of endorphins, the body's herbal painkillers, reflexology can advantage the favored stimulation.

Notably, reflexology now not handiest gives bodily advantages, however it may moreover beautify highbrow and emotional health by lowering pressure and promoting relaxation.

People who be afflicted by persistent pressure or anxiety can discover reflexology specially beneficial as it could assist them experience greater snug and comfortable.

The gastric and airway systems, among others, can be specially targeted by using reflexology to beautify their fashionable health and capability.

Furthermore, reflexology can stimulate the reflex factors on the toes that correspond to the adrenal glands and extremely good areas of the frame related to stress and emotion, making it superb for mood and emotional nicely-being.

Reflexology can useful resource human beings in retaining their enjoy of equilibrium and top health amidst the stresses of each day existence, specially in mild of the pressures of present day society.

In precis, reflexology is a secure and effective remedy to take into account for people trying to beautify their health and properly-being.

With a balanced mixture of perplexity and burstiness, reflexology offers a holistic method to decreasing stress, assuaging ache, and enhancing precise organs and structures within the frame.

As a herbal desire for boosting fashionable health and exquisite of lifestyles, reflexology gives various blessings and huge-ranging programs.

HOW REFLEXOLOGY WORKS

Reflexology, an opportunity therapeutic modality, includes the utility of stress to particular points on the ft, hands, and ears.

It is idea that those factors correspond to excellent organs and structures inside the body, and via using manipulating them, reflexologists intention to instill tranquility, decrease ache, and decorate holistic nicely-being. But how does this enigmatic exercise function?

Despite its big use, the mechanics underlying reflexology are however largely unknown, but, numerous theories had been located out to provide an cause at the back of its outcomes.

One of these theories indicates that reflexology operates with the aid of way of evoking the frame's inherent restoration capacities.

By using strain to pick factors at the ft, palms, or ears, reflexologists also can activate the aggravating tool and increase blood go with the flow to various regions of the body.

This can also aid in mitigating ache, ameliorating infection, and inducing rest and remarkable affect.

Another concept is that reflexology works thru restoring equilibrium to the body's energy systems.

A latest community of power channels known as meridians is idea to manipulate the frame in conventional Chinese treatment.

When those meridians end up obstructed or disrupted, they will initiate physical and emotional disturbances.

Reflexologists attempt to unclog the ones channels and harmonize the frame's power structures with the aid of way of focused on particular reflex elements.

A 1/three hypothesis is that reflexology operates by using way of the use of inciting the discharge of endorphins and specific natural analgesics.

Endorphins are endogenous chemical substances which could mitigate pain and engender emotions of contentment.

Reflexologists may additionally additionally elicit the release of endorphins by means of using the usage of manipulating nice reflex elements, thereby attenuating ache and fostering relaxation.

A further concept proposes that reflexology stimulates the body's lymphatic machine.

This device is liable for putting off waste products from the frame and preventing infections.

Chapter 21: The Reflexology Map

Reflexology, a recovery technique that applies strain to particular elements at the feet, hands, and ears, is thought to correspond with specific organs and systems inside the body, in line with the principle that there are reflex regions on the ones elements of the body which is probably linked to the frame's power pathways.

These reflex areas may be stimulated to sell restoration and balance, which makes reflexology a unique exercise for maintaining top-first-rate health and properly-being.

The Reflexology Map, an essential device for reflexologists, outlines the reflex elements at the ft, arms, and ears, making it much less hard for practitioners to become aware about which areas to interest on all through a consultation.

Ten zones, each representing a one-of-a-kind body element, are marked on the map. Zone 1 represents the head and neck, at the same time as Zone 5 represents the reproductive organs.

The map moreover has factors, inclusive of these for the renal device, liver, and lungs, that represent unique organs alongside those zones.

By making use of strain to the ones elements, reflexologists can sell the float of electricity and blood to the ones organs, which can decorate their function.

The Reflexology Map is likewise useful for individuals interested by self-reflexology.

With this map, humans can carry out self-reflexology thru making use of pressure to the reflex factors on the feet, fingers, or ears to promote recovery and stability within the body.

The Reflexology Map isn't always best a clean diagram of reflex factors however a crucial device that promotes the flow of power and blood in some unspecified time in the destiny of the frame.

Reflexology practitioners are capable to utilize it to pinpoint areas that ought to be handled to cope with unique health conditions, which embody migraines, digestive problems, or stress.

It is a complicated track of response websites that map to numerous sections of the body.

By the use of the map to find out the reflex points that correspond to particular health problems, human beings can also sell recuperation and stability of their our bodies.

In forestall, the Reflexology Map is a useful device for both reflexologists and those interested in self-reflexology.

With its ten zones and unique elements that correspond to organs, the map permits practitioners to promote restoration and balance in the frame by means of stimulating the reflex regions on the feet, fingers, and ears.

By facts the standards of reflexology and the usage of the map to select out the reflex elements that correspond to big components of the frame, people can hold maximum nice fitness and nicely-being.

REFLEXOLOGY FOR

PROMOTING HEALTH

Reflexology is a holistic modality that includes the use of stress and massage techniques on unique areas of the feet, hands, and ears to sell everyday fitness and well-being.

Reflex net web sites on the frame that correspond to severa sections are inspired in some unspecified time in the future of this opportunity treatment, which has been verified to enhance flow into, assist the immune machine, and motive the body's inborn recovery mechanisms.

The primary mechanism with the aid of which reflexology promotes ordinary health and properly-being is through improving motion.

Reflexologists believe that via stimulating the reflex factors at the ft, fingers, and ears, they're capable of increase blood go together with the glide and oxygen to the corresponding organs and tissues.

This advanced float can also moreover beneficial resource in decreasing infection, enhancing immunological reaction, and accelerating the restoration method.

Additionally, improved flow into can help to ease stress and sell relaxation, each of which could gain full-size health.

Furthermore, reflexology is concept to prompt the self-recovery mechanisms of the frame via stress carried out to specific reflex elements, thereby promoting the body's herbal recuperation strategies.

This enables cope with a number of illnesses with the beneficial aid of selling the frame's capability to heal itself, from persistent pain to digestive issues.

Reflexology can also reduce the need for medicinal pills or exclusive interventions by way of promoting the body's herbal restoration strategies, which may be excessive terrific for human beings looking for a extra herbal technique to health and well being.

Reflexology is moreover a fulfillment at encouraging relaxation and decreasing strain, both of which have a large impact on preferred fitness and well-being.

When someone is beneath strain, cortisol is created, and it's far dangerous to great biological methods similarly to the immune device.

By promoting rest, reflexology can assist to reduce cortisol degrees, that can decorate immune feature, reduce infection, and sell recovery.

Reflexology also can help humans revel in peaceful and snug, that can improve their mood and reduce depressive and worrying mind.

Finally, reflexology is a complementary treatment that would assist unique treatments and interventions.

For instance, it may be used along conventional scientific treatments to promote recovery and reduce aspect effects.

To decorate its outcomes and boom favored fitness and nicely-being, it can moreover be used with other complementary treatments like rub down or acupuncture.

Reflexologists can provide an included technique for health and properly-being that covers the mental, non secular, and physical aspects of health thru way of taking part with special healthcare experts.

REFLEXOLOGY FOR

RELIEVING TENSION

Reflexology is a complementary remedy that includes making use of stress to specific factors on the ft, arms, or ears to stimulate the body's herbal recuperation reaction.

This remedy is rooted inside the principle that those reflex factors are linked to numerous organs, glands, and tremendous factors of the frame via strength pathways.

By focused on the ones reflex factors, reflexology can help to spark off the body's herbal healing mechanisms, that would promote fundamental fitness and health.

One way reflexology can assist to alleviate anxiety and strain is thru the usage of selling relaxation.

Through the software program of pressure to the reflex elements, tension is launched, and a sense of relaxation permeates the body.

This rest reaction is connected to a drop in stress hormones like cortisol, that could extensively decorate fitness in elegant and offset the unfavourable effects pressure has at the body.

Moreover, reflexology can boost blood waft and oxygenation within the muscle agencies and tissues that are tormented by tension, which allows to lower infection and alleviate ache, due to this enhancing mobility.

The growth in flow into also promotes recovery, making it a valuable tool for those experiencing persistent ache and different related conditions.

Beyond its bodily advantages, reflexology is likewise beneficial in selling intellectual and emotional nicely-being.

By inducing relaxation and decreasing stress, reflexology can enhance mood and reduce tension and despair.

An full-size development in life amazing and an popular feeling of balance outcomes from this emotional and intellectual health.

In end, reflexology is a valuable tool in stopping tension and stress at the same time as improving famous health and nicely-being.

Through the targeted pressure implemented to specific reflex elements, reflexology can spark off the body's natural restoration mechanisms, stimulate blood go together with the float and oxygenation, and sell intellectual and emotional well-being.

Thus, reflexology can function a stable and effective complementary treatment for humans experiencing tension or strain.

REFLEXOLOGY FOR

ELIMINATING ANXIETY

The exercise of reflexology is predicated upon the essential intention of firing up the neurons which may be intricately associated with the fearful device, spinal twine, and adrenal glands.

This is finished through manner of the use of centered strain to sure areas of the palms, feet, and ears.

Reflexology has acquired popularity as an opportunity treatment for pressure and tension-related conditions.

By manipulating the ones connections within the body, the ensuing results can produce regulation of the body's automatic skills, further to cut fee in tension and merchandising of rest.

The important involvement of the worried device is one properly-cited element of the intellectual and bodily consequences of pressure, which include tension.

Studies display that pressure triggers cortisol launch from the body, that would show risky if publicity persists.

However, through stimulation of the reflex factors related to the autonomic apprehensive system – governing automated capabilities including respiration, coronary heart price, and digestion.

Reflexology has the potential to regulate and restore balance in the apprehensive machine.

In reaction to pressure, the adrenal glands release chemical substances which incorporates adrenaline and cortisol.

Chapter 22: Reflexology For Losing Weight

Reflexology, an ancient practice that employs using strain factors at the ft, fingers, and ears, has been gaining traction as a herbal and powerful approach to facilitate weight loss.

By activating reflex elements that correspond to the digestive system and metabolism, reflexology has the capability to regulate hormones, beautify metabolic characteristic, and enhance digestion.

By integrating reflexology proper right right into a weight loss regimen, you can likely expand the efficacy of the program and provide prolonged-term weight manipulate useful resource.

The intimate connection some of the digestive device and metabolism makes them vital problems for any weight loss assignment.

By controlling hormones which may be crucial for metabolism and starvation, including leptin, cortisol, and insulin, reflexology might also moreover assist people shed pounds.

By stimulating reflex factors on the feet that correspond to the pancreas, thyroid, and adrenal glands, reflexology can modify these hormones and promote a healthful metabolic fee, it definitely is conducive to weight loss.

Every weight loss normal ought to correctly deal with digestion.

Reflexology can promote digestion thru stimulating reflex elements on the feet that correspond to the stomach, intestines, and colon, facilitating extended blood waft and oxygen supply to the digestive system.

Reflexology can also alleviate digestive issues which incorporates constipation and bloating that may obstruct weight loss development.

Stress is a essential factor that may inhibit weight reduction improvement.

Reflexology can help reduce strain levels through using the usage of selling relaxation and lowering cortisol levels.

By stimulating reflex factors at the feet that correspond to the worried tool, reflexology can decrease pressure degrees, potentially selling weight loss and famous well-being.

The incorporation of reflexology proper right into a healthy eating plan can assist optimize the effectiveness of this gadget and provide prolonged-time period weight control manual.

Reflexology can help adjust hormones, enhance digestion, lessen pressure levels, and promote relaxation - all of which may be essential additives of weight reduction.

Reflexology is a high-quality addition to any weight loss program or exercise ordinary while you maintain in mind that it is a non-invasive, steady, and all-herbal technique to assist weight reduction.

REFLEXOLOGY FOR REDUCING PAIN

Reflexology is an ancient herbal restoration remedy that has been implemented for masses of years to alleviate ache and beautify regular nicely being.

Reflex spots discovered on the palms, ft, and ears are said to connect with numerous frame elements, that is the idea for this treatment's important idea.

By stimulating those reflex elements, therapists can efficiently restrict ache and tension in the affected areas of the frame, along side the lower lower back or neck.

The art of reflexology is renowned for its unheard of capability to instigate relaxation and reduce stress ranges.

The underlying mechanisms contain the release of anxiety within the muscle agencies through the induction of profound rest, which could mitigate ache and provide alleviation from ache in high-quality components of the frame.

The multifaceted and complicated blessings of reflexology moreover embody enhancing flow into, that can useful resource in preventing the horrible impact of pollution that acquire within the frame, inflicting ache and contamination.

This is possible through the stimulation of reflex factors placed at the toes, arms, and ears that could counteract the construct-up of pollutants, thereby lessening the burden of pain and contamination in affected areas of the frame.

Another manner reflexology can relieve pain is by way of triggering the release of endorphins that function as herbal painkillers generated via the frame.

Endorphins are produced with the useful resource of the frame on every occasion it endures sensations of soreness like pain so one can assist the body control those emotions.

Reflexology acts by way of the usage of inducing the manufacturing of endorphins, which could substantially lessen pain and enhance present day well being.

In addition to its already superb variety of advantages, reflexology has been determined to beautify the immune system.

A reinforced immune device can higher equip the body to fend off infections and ailments.

Reflexology can assist to beautify the immune device through invigorating the lymphatic device, which acts as a purifier, disposing of pollutants and waste cloth from the frame, thereby improving regular health and decreasing pain levels.

Overall, reflexology is an immensely efficacious and natural remedy which can drastically reduce ache and improve general health.

The stimulation of reflex elements located on the feet, hands, and ears can foster rest, enhance motion, stimulate endorphin production, and beautify the immune device.

Reflexology should turn out to be a absolutely first-rate desire in case you're looking for a natural technique to lessen pain and decorate your today's health.

REFLEXOLOGY FOR

HEADACHES AND MIGRAINES

Reflexology, a non-invasive treatment, is a natural technique that includes utilising stress to precise reflex factors on the fingers, feet, and ears.

These factors are related to numerous organs, glands, and body elements and may beautify blood go with the drift and electricity float at the same time as stimulated.

The standard health and properly-being of the body can gain from this exercise, with headaches and migraines being some of the ailments reflexology can beneficial useful resource.

The large toe houses one of the handiest reflex factors for treating complications and migraines.

This reflex trouble corresponds to the top and may be activated via applying stress to its base.

This reflex factor may be stimulated to reduce headache and migraine ache and discomfort, improve blood waft, and relieve head and neck strain.

Middle and ring arms include powerful reflex factors that correspond to the top and may assist relieve tension through the use of strain to their bases.

Additionally, such stimulation might possibly encourage tranquility, relaxation, and infection bargain, which may lessen headaches and migraines.

Another effective reflex aspect is located in the webbing a number of the thumb and index finger.

This reflex component corresponds to the neck and may be activated with the useful resource of using pressure to the region.

Activation of this reflex point can lower neck tension and decorate blood circulate, thereby alleviating the signs and symptoms and signs and symptoms and signs and symptoms of headaches and migraines.

Reflexology furthermore aids in relieving sinus complications because of sinus infection and congestion.

Stimulation of the reflex factors on the toes and toes just like the sinuses can reduce infection and encourage drainage, main to symptom relief.

In stop, reflexology is a natural remedy that may correctly address headaches and migraines via stimulating the reflex elements just like the top and neck.

By improving blood float, lowering anxiety and irritation, and promoting relaxation, reflexology offers a stable, non-invasive remedy alternative for people searching out treatment from their signs and symptoms and signs and symptoms.

REFLEXOLOGY FOR INSOMNIA

Reflexology, an possibility therapy that employs stress on the toes, fingers, and ears to alleviate ache and promote rest, has a wealth of blessings.

Among them, it could enhance sleep first-rate via activating precise reflex factors that correspond to the worrying and endocrine systems, in the end decreasing stress and anxiety, and inducing a state of calm and relaxation that fosters restful sleep.

Numerous physical physiological abilties, which consist of sleep, are tightly managed with the useful resource of the neurological tool.

Reflex points that align with the anxious tool are placed on the feet, and making use of stress to those elements can offer a calming effect to each the frame and thoughts, lowering anxiety tiers and placing the extent for rest.

As a end end result, it turns into easier to nod off and stay asleep and the quality of your sleep improves.

By generating melatonin, which conjures up tiredness, the endocrine device in addition performs a giant feature in the control of sleep.

Reflexology can prompt the reflex factors that relate to the endocrine machine, helping inside the law of hormone degrees and boosting sleep first-class, making it especially beneficial for those with insomnia or unique sleep issues.

Reflexology is likewise capable of selling rest by means of the use of way of growing blood go along with the go with the glide and oxygenation at a few stage within the frame, a phenomenon that complements glide and decreases muscle tension, fostering a sensation of calm and tranquility that is particularly useful for selling restful sleep.

On the whole, reflexology is an definitely regular and non-invasive technique that could beautify rest and beautify sleep exceptional by way of triggering reflex factors related to the worried and endocrine systems.

Whether employed on my own or in tandem with extraordinary relaxation strategies, reflexology has a awesome capability for facilitating restorative, invigorating sleep, and improving generic fitness and properly-being.

Chapter 23: Reflexology For Digestive Issues

Reflexology, an unintrusive and complete modality, encompasses the workout of exerting stress on notable reflex factors on the hands, ears, or toes.

As a end result, it turns on and encourages the capability of corresponding organs, glands, and structures, which restores balance and promotes healing.

Reflexology's effectiveness is maximum absolutely validated within the remedy of several digestive issues, which includes indigestion, bloating, and constipation.

Constipation, a pervasive hassle that a multitude of humans confront, can discover comfort with reflexology.

Reflexologists can observe pressure at the reflex points at the toes that align with the rectum and colon to prompt bowel motion and alleviate constipation.

Furthermore, reflexology serves as an splendid device to mitigate the tension and pressure that commonly exacerbates digestive ailments.

Another triumphing digestive hassle, bloating, stems from severa elements, which incorporates impaired digestion, intolerances, and stress.

Reflexology gives a promising alternative in phrases of improving digestion and pressure cut price, thereby mitigating bloating.

With the stimulation of the reflex factors at the ft that relate to the belly, small gut, and colon, reflexology allows stronger digestive feature and minimizes bloating and fuel.

Indigestion, any other tough and continual digestive contamination, can be alleviated with reflexology.

Poor food plan, gastrointestinal maladies, and stress are maximum of the myriad of reasons for indigestion.

By stimulating the reflex elements at the ft that correspond to the liver, belly, pancreas, and gallbladder, reflexology can decorate digestive characteristic and reduce indigestion.

The cease quit end result is a extra entire technique that addresses the underlying motive while promoting better digestive fitness.

Moreover, reflexology contributes to the enhancement of digestive function, the bargain of infection, and the advertising and advertising and marketing of healing through stimulating the reflex factors that correspond to the digestive device.

Reflexology's potential to lessen stress, a time-commemorated motive for severa digestive issues, similarly bolsters its effectiveness.

In end, reflexology is a completely a success method for treating digestive issues like indigestion, bloating, and constipation.

Through the stimulation of the reflex elements that correspond to the digestive gadget, reflexology improves digestive feature, reduces contamination, and promotes restoration.

Those suffering from digestive issues need to recall reflexology as a steady and feasible restoration possibility.

REFLEXOLOGY FOR

MENSTRUAL PROLEMS

Reflexology, an historic holistic recuperation modality, deploys centered pressure on specific elements placed on the toes, hands, and ears, triggering neural pathways and enhancing blood motion to numerous organs and tissues within the frame.

To assuage menstrual issues, reflexology employs the stimulation of reflex factors that correspond to the reproductive system.

These reflex elements can be placed on the inner arch of the foot and require targeted pressure to enhance blood waft to reproductive organs.

Reflexology correctly recovery procedures various menstrual troubles, collectively with bleeding excessively, period inconsistencies, and symptoms of PMS, similarly to assisting in controlling the cycle of menstruation.

Hormone imbalances and PMS signs and signs may be treated via the use of way of stimulating adrenal gland, pituitary gland, and thyroid gland reflex elements located at the toes.

Stress and anxiety, which act as aggravators for menstrual troubles, can be quelled through activating reflex elements that correspond to the apprehensive tool, as a result reaching a country of frame tranquility.

All in all, reflexology, with its non-invasive and danger loose approach, emerges as a reliable possibility recuperation technique to mitigate menstrual difficulties.

By inducing the reflex factors related to the reproductive system, endocrine system, and worried device, reflexology affords girls an effective, herbal remedy option that lets in balance hormones, mitigate pain and stress, alter menstrual drift, and provide numerous unique blessings.

Should you come across menstrual problems, reflexology represents a possible remedy desire that merits your careful interest.

REFLEXOLOGY FOR

RESPIRATORY ISSUES

Reflexology, an ancient complementary remedy, involves making use of stress to precise reflex factors on the palms, feet, and ears, promoting healing and mitigating ache.

This holistic modality, with its roots in conventional remedy, has examined effective over centuries, treating a big kind of conditions, together with folks who implicate the breathing device.

Take bronchial allergic reactions, a continual respiratory scenario plaguing tens of loads of thousands worldwide, for example.

It triggers airway contamination, essential to mucous manufacturing, and motives an obstructed air passage.

Yet, by the use of the usage of stimulating corresponding reflex elements at the bronchial tubes and lungs, reflexology can enhance airflow and reduce inflammation, alleviating the ensuing respiration troubles.

But allergies is not the most effective respiratory hassle that reflexology can address.

Bronchitis is each other commonplace ailment that reflexology can relieve.

Marked via bronchial tubes' contamination, bronchitis activates an uncongenial cough, wheezing, and respiration impediments.

However, reflexology can alleviate these signs and symptoms via using triggering reflex factors related to the respiratory device, the lungs, and bronchial tubes.

Better but, reflexology can beautify circulate, cut down inflammation, and foster restoration, all of that may ease ache and soothe breathing issues.

Reflexology not simplest has health advantages for the frame but furthermore for the thoughts and the spirit.

For instance, pressure and worry can exacerbate the signs and symptoms of hypersensitive reactions and bronchitis, making them tremendously more hard to govern.

However, reflexology can alleviate stress and anxiety, promoting rest, and improving temper, which can have a big impact on the general wonderful of life for respiratory hassle sufferers.

It permits them control symptoms greater efficaciously and promotes superior fitness and properly-being.

In conclusion, reflexology is a secure and efficacious complementary treatment for treating respiration problems collectively with hypersensitive reactions and bronchitis.

By stimulating reflex elements associated with the respiratory device, reflexology can decorate respiration, lessen irritation, and alleviate one of a kind symptoms.

Reflexology can also beautify widespread emotional and highbrow fitness via encouraging rest, reducing anxiety and tension, and distinctive blessings.

These blessings make reflexology a valuable tool in handling respiration troubles and selling favored fitness and nicely-being.

REFLEXOLOGY FOR

THE IMMUNE SYSTEM

Reflexology, an possibility restoration technique, includes the application of strain to precise elements at the arms, feet, or ears that correspond to various organs and structures within the frame.

The results of reflexology on the immune gadget are notable. It impacts the immune gadget favorably through stimulating the reflex elements related to the spleen and lymphatic machine.

In addition to its immune-boosting houses, reflexology can facilitate the removal of waste and pollutants from the frame through using improving lymphatic go with the flow and characteristic.

Given the lymphatic device's critical characteristic in retaining immunity, reflexology can feature an effective modality for activating this device.

Along similar strains, reflexology can red meat up the immune system's resilience via augmenting the manufacturing of white blood cells and bolstering the body's safety mechanisms in opposition to infections and sicknesses.

Reflexology's capacity in mitigating strain and selling relaxation can further augment its immunity-improving homes.

Stress has prolonged been recognized as an immunosuppressive agent, and reflexology's ability to counteract that is noteworthy.

By lowering strain, reflexology can beautify the immune tool's characteristic, increase flow into, and promote average fitness and nicely-being.

Moreover, reflexology's capacity to enhance circulate is vital to its immunomodulatory consequences.

Efficient movement is critical for transporting vital vitamins and oxygen ultimately of the frame and getting rid of dangerous waste and pollutants.

Chapter 24: Reflexology For

PREGNANCY AND CHILDBIRTH

Reflexology, a complementary treatment that is garnering increasing reputation amongst expectant mothers, entails using stress to particular elements on the feet, hands, or ears that correspond to brilliant organs and systems inside the frame.

By reducing strain and anxiety, reflexology can aid in getting ready the frame for childbirth at the same time as additionally alleviating some of the discomforts of pregnancy.

Here are five strategies wherein reflexology may be beneficial for pregnant women.

Firstly, reflexology can promote rest and alleviate stress.

Pregnancy can be an extremely annoying time, and reflexology can assist pregnant women to unwind and loosen up.

Reflexology, which dreams the neurological device, can lessen tension and foster calmness, which may be particularly useful for those who enjoy tension or disappointment at some stage in being pregnant.

Secondly, reflexology can offer consolation from once more ache.

The lower again may additionally enjoy great pressure due to the truth the infant grows, resulting in discomfort and ache.

However, reflexology can in particular aim the reflex factors in the toes that correspond to the lower lower back, imparting remedy from pain and tension.

Regular reflexology periods can also enhance posture and prevent again ache from becoming a continual hassle.

Thirdly, reflexology can useful resource digestion and ease constipation.

Constipation, fuel, and bloating are not unusual digestive troubles that pregnant girls come upon.

By concentrated on the reflex factors that correspond to the digestive machine, reflexology can help to alleviate those signs and signs and improve digestion.

This may be especially useful for the ones experiencing those issues because of hormonal adjustments or nutritional modifications subsequently of pregnancy.

Fourthly, reflexology can sell restful sleep.

Due to pain, anxiety, or hormonal changes, many expectant mothers battle to get adequate sleep.

Reflexology can promote relaxation and beautify the satisfactory of sleep through the usage of way of stimulating the reflex factors that correspond to the worried machine.

Regular reflexology intervals can help expectant mothers to reap the relaxation they require to sense revitalized and wholesome.

Finally, reflexology can prepare the frame for childbirth.

By stimulating the reflex points that correspond to the reproductive device, reflexology can assist to prepared the frame for tough work and shipping.

Furthermore, through selling rest and lowering strain stages, reflexology can improve women's self warranty and sense of empowerment for the duration of childbirth.

In end, reflexology may be a constant and effective approach for alleviating the discomforts of pregnancy and getting ready the frame for childbirth.

By specializing in particular reflex factors within the ft, palms, or ears, reflexology can reduce stress, relieve pain, enhance digestion, promote restful sleep, and equipped the body for hard paintings and delivery.

Pregnant girls interested by reflexology must are looking for recommendation from an authorized reflexologist to talk about their problems and treatment targets.

BEST REFLEXOLOGY TECHNIQUES

Reflexology, a recuperation approach with roots in ancient instances, consists of making use of stress to unique elements at the toes, arms, and ears to inspire the frame's herbal recuperation techniques and beautify massive well-being.

There are numerous strategies for appearing reflexology, every presenting its precise set of benefits.

Some of the simplest embody the thumb-on foot method, the greedy and backup method, the sun plexus reflexology technique, the lymph node drainage reflexology method, and the vertebral twist reflexology approach.

The thumb-walking method, for example, is a useful approach for undertaking relaxation, relieving ache, reducing pressure, and enhancing glide.

A therapist applies strain to focused regions using their thumbs, frequently developing the depth as required.

This method is specially beneficial for human beings with chronic pain or tension, or the ones trying to find a chilled impact.

The grasping and backup approach, which makes use of arms to apply stress to unique factors at the feet or hands, is particularly effective in stimulating reflex factors related to the digestive and lymphatic structures.

A therapist hooks their fingers at some stage in the foot or hand, applies pressure to the favored region, releases it, and repeats the method numerous instances.

The sun plexus reflexology method involves applying organization strain to the solar plexus reflex factor positioned within the center of the foot, that is in particular powerful for lowering pressure and selling rest, enhancing digestion, and boosting the immune device.

The therapist repeats this way numerous instances, freeing stress in between.

The lymphatic drainage reflexology method stimulates the lymphatic device, answerable for getting rid of pollutants and waste products from the body.

A therapist applies mild strain to the lymphatic reflex elements located at the toes or fingers, promoting the glide of lymphatic fluid and improving simple health.

This remedy may be very useful for human beings with edema or other clinical conditions that harm the lymphatic machine.

Finally, the vertebral twist reflexology method, which incorporates the use of arms to use pressure to specific elements alongside the spine, is fantastically effective in reducing anxiety, enhancing glide, promoting rest, and reducing pressure.

The therapist applies strain to the backbone, gently twisting it to release anxiety and enhance movement.

This technique is specially useful for human beings with lower back ache or awesome spinal situations.

In give up, reflexology gives a stable and powerful manner to sell not unusual fitness, relieve pressure, and reduce tension.

With severa techniques to be had, a informed reflexologist can tailor their treatment to the particular dreams of their clients, incorporating numerous techniques including the thumb-on foot technique, the greedy and backup method, the sun plexus reflexology approach, the lymphatic drainage reflexology approach, and the vertebral twist reflexology method.

BEST REFLEXOLOGY TREATMENTS

Reflexology is a highly ultra-modern and complicated holistic recovery exercising that entails the skillful software of stress to unique reflex factors positioned at the toes, palms, and ears.

This remedy is founded at the fundamental principle that every organ and device inside the body possesses a corresponding reflex factor on both the feet, palms, or ears.

By utilising this profound knowledge, reflexology treatments can provide an intensive variety of compelling blessings, in conjunction with however not restricted to lowering strain and anxiety, selling move, fortifying the immune device, and invigorating everyday properly-being.

In this concept-horrifying article, we're able to find out the best reflexology treatments that can help you enjoy honestly cushty, revitalized, and refreshed.

The first and essential reflexology treatment that we quite recommend is foot reflexology, that may be a definitely transformative experience that includes the clever software software of stress to precise reflex elements positioned at the feet that correspond to various organs and structures inside the course of the frame.

Foot reflexology is an super and fantastically efficacious remedy alternative that might assist alleviate strain and anxiety within the ft, invigorate circulate, and promote deep rest at some point of the entire body.

It is a superior remedy choice, specially for folks who spend prolonged durations status or be stricken with the aid of plantar fasciitis or foot ache.

The second out of the normal reflexology treatment that we enthusiastically advocate is hand reflexology, that is a sophisticated remedy that consists of skillfully making use of strain to precise reflex factors positioned at the fingers that correspond to various organs and systems within the body.

Chapter 25: Beyond Reflexology

Reflexology, an possibility healing modality that is characterized through the use of the software of strain to unique elements at the fingers, toes, and ears, is a pretty bendy art that can be synergistically combined with an array of different practices to benefit an higher recuperation very last results.

One such artwork this is regularly conjoined with reflexology is aromatherapy, a healing method that harnesses the benefits of important oils to enhance the relaxation and calming consequences of reflexology, primary to a profound betterment of every bodily and emotional properly-being.

In addition to having an effect on the body, the aroma of the oils can also spark off the smell glands, that would further beautify the general healing manner.

Meditation is some other art work that can be mixed with reflexology, and masses of discover that once applied in tandem, reflexology and meditation can useful resource in accomplishing a deeper us of a of rest and intellectual readability.

The interaction of the two techniques fosters a deeper feeling of harmony and stability in each factor of one's life.

In addition to aromatherapy and meditation, reflexology also can be paired with song remedy to sell rest and increase the restoration way.

Soft, mellow melodies can assist lessen pressure, anxiety, and melancholy, even as simultaneously promoting physical and emotional recuperation.

The affects of music can also excite the brain, inflicting the endorphins—natural painkillers and temper boosters—to be released.

Moreover, reflexology may be synergistically blended with yoga, a holistic workout that entails a series of poses and stretches that might help improve circulate, lessen tension, and promote rest.

When blended with reflexology, yoga can heighten the recuperation advantages of every practices, enhancing flexibility, balance, and ordinary physical nicely-being.

Reflexology has a promising destiny because of the fact that extra people are turning to different strategies to beautify their physical and highbrow fitness.

It is pretty in all likelihood that reflexology will preserve to gain reputation as a recognized kind of remedy as greater studies on its benefits is undertaken.

Furthermore, advances in generation may additionally bring about improved accessibility to reflexology for those who live in a long way off or underserved areas.

Reflexology is predicted to benefit popularity over the imminent years due to the truth to the developing name for for holistic and opportunity treatment alternatives.

Chapter 26: Who Is Reflexology For?

Reflexology has installed to be powerful within the remedy of a huge sort of pathologies. For example, acupuncture and different techniques successfully deal with such illnesses as:

Illnesses of the musculoskeletal system;

fearful issues (neuritis, neurosis, neuralgia, insomnia, depression, migraine, VSD, stuttering, and so on.);

put up-demanding conditions;

cardiovascular ailment;

conditions after strokes;

ailments of the genitourinary machine;

sexual problems;

respiratory diseases;

ENT pathology, SARS, acute respiratory infections;

endocrine pathologies, hormonal problems ;

metabolic disorders, obese;

allergic ailments ;

sicknesses of the digestive device ;

craving for smoking, and so on.

Reflexology isn't always indicated for the following conditions:

oncopathology;

blood clotting issues;

severe coronary heart failure ;

extreme renal failure ;

infectious and pores and skin illnesses in the acute diploma;

acute intellectual issues;

kids and vintage age;

being pregnant, lactation.

Before making a decision to recommend or restriction reflexology techniques, the doctor ought to speak with the affected individual, have a take a look at the overall medical image of his contamination, and person trends.

Neurologists, reflexologists of our sanatorium are proficient in all traditional and current-day strategies of diagnosing and treating neurological illnesses, which includes strategies of reflex remedy.

Acupuncture strategies and other sorts of acupressure allow reflexologists to deal with sicknesses of severa etiology and severity, reaching a solid and prolonged-lasting impact. A kind of restoration strategies makes reflexology to be had to almost any class of patients.

In the complex treatment of ache, we use acupuncture. The health practitioner-reflexologist who owns all of the techniques of reflexology, has the brilliant qualification beauty, and has again and again been professional in reflexology, consults, and conducts treatment.

Acupuncture is the introduction of specific needles into sure regions of the pores and pores and skin and underlying tissues for the reason of prophylactic or recovery consequences on the frame. Acupuncture is used to cope with sicknesses followed via pain and infection. This method is widely used for the remedy of osteochondrosis, neuritis, neurology, menopausal syndrome, migraines, insomnia, all over again ache, in the liver, and awesome pain syndromes.

One of the strategies of acupuncture - electroreflexotherapy, is widely used to cope with neurasthenia, melancholy, infertility, Raynaud's syndrome, weight problems, arterial excessive blood strain, the pain of unknown etiology, and masses of different illnesses.

Indications for remedy:

osteocondritis of the spine;

neuralgia of the trigeminal and facial nerves, listening to loss;

vegetovascular dystonia;

insomnia;

migraine;

persistent fatigue;

neuroses, tics;

allergy;

smoking.

The fundamental warning symptoms for the use of reflexology:

ailments of the musculoskeletal tool (arthrosis, arthritis, osteochondrosis, herniated discs);

ailments of the aggravating tool and psycho-emotional problems (neuralgia, neuritis, migraine, despair, neurosis, chronic fatigue, sexual disease not because of organic problems);

pains of numerous etiology and localization (headache, dental, postoperative, and so on.);

ailments of the cardiovascular device (IHD, obliterating endarteritis, arterial high blood pressure, vegetovascular asthenia) ;

pores and pores and pores and skin ailments (urticaria, dermatitis, eczema, psoriasis, neurodermatitis);

respiratory sicknesses (bronchitis, pneumonia, bronchial bronchial bronchial bronchial asthma);

hypersensitivity;

illnesses of the digestive tool (gastritis, peptic ulcer, liver illness, pancreatitis, cholecystitis, colitis);

illnesses of ENT organs (otitis media, rhinitis, sinusitis, laryngitis);

illnesses of the urogenital organs (pyelonephritis, cystitis, prostatitis, reduced performance, enuresis);

gynecological illnesses (persistent inflammatory illnesses, menstrual issues, menopause);

diseases of the endocrine gadget and metabolic disorders (weight problems, diabetes mellitus, and its complications, female hormonal troubles);

sleep troubles;

tobacco addiction.

List of stylish contraindications for reflexology.

All sicknesses are in the extreme level, continual sicknesses are in the stage of decompensation.

Infectious and venereal illnesses in acute or contagious form.

All kinds of tuberculosis are inside the lively degree.

Chapter 27: Foot Rubdown

Foot massage has been used in view that ancient times through Eastern peoples as a technique to lighten up, cope with many sicknesses and keep health in big. There are about 70 thousand nerve endings at the foot, through which the foot is set up with all inner organs. Leg and foot rub down is an incomparable satisfaction, which no longer only relieves worn-out toes, tones the muscles of the legs and the entire frame, however is likewise a completely specific amusing manner.

Indeed, foot rub down is a very, very excellent pastime that consequences inside the rebirth, if now not of the entire organism, then at the least of the forces as an entire. A leg and foot rub down is a chunk considered one among a type from, say, a lower again rub down. The distinction is that when massaging the ft and legs, now not handiest the muscle tissues themselves are stimulated, which may be affected, however a useful impact is exerted at the whole frame foot massage.

And the purpose for that is a massive variety of reflex factors which might be responsible for the kingdom of the body as an entire. So, as an example, inside the arch of the foot, there can be a huge attention of factors, which in cutting-edge reflexology are correlated with the backbone. Therefore, stimulation of this vicinity of the foot will help relieve lower once more ache, bring preferred consolation to the frame.

Stimulation of the ft has a useful effect at the eyes, ears, enamel, and gums, and sinuses. Do you keep in thoughts how in formative years, even as you had a chilly, your grandmother rubbed your ft with vodka, and mainly every finger, and then the following morning the cold receded, your nostril started to respire more freely, and your eyes stopped watering?

On the identical points positioned on the plantar a part of the foot, in huge, you can write an entire Talmud - there are factors that correspond to the internal organs, great well-being, or perhaps the temper of a person.

Active have an impact on on those elements consequences in an improvement in general nicely-being and the elimination of numerous pains.

Chinese medication medical doctors say that foot rub down is actually all that a person needs for happiness. After all, if you test the format of acupuncture factors at the ft, we are able to see projections of all organs and structures of the human frame there. Do you've got got have been given spinal issues? Take care of the lower decrease back of the foot. Stuffy nose? Excuse me - massage of the toes will save you from problem.

There aren't such lots of perpendiculars inside the human frame, or alternatively, excellent one. This is the foot, the only a part of our frame this is perpendicular to all super elements of it. Foot rub down has been referred to to people on the grounds that historical times. According to the thoughts of ancient Indian and Chinese medical doctors, whose views and practices have now not misplaced their relevance even these days, the notice of electricity flows intersecting in the foot is simply vast. A lot of foot receptors will let you effect nearly all human organs.

Doing a foot massage, you mobilize your power, boom the tone of the whole organism. The correct effect at the foot will assist to do away with or alleviate a whole lot of painful phenomena. But except this restoration characteristic, foot massage has a totally extraordinary impact on the emotional us of a.

Foot rubdown can without trouble relieve strain and enhance temper. No surprise the ancient sages recommended to rubdown the ft to repair no longer best internal harmony however moreover to enhance verbal exchange with the out of doors international, which changed into pondered in numerous ancient treatises. Modern medication, no matter some "careful" attitude to the training of the ancients, even though acknowledges the beneficial effects of foot rubdown, each on the general state of affairs of the frame and character organs.

The effect on the energy points located at the feet gives awesome consequences. After all, each nerve completing is inextricably related with our certainly one of a type organs. For instance, the thumb is accountable for the pinnacle, and the middle and index fingers are for the eyes. Foot rub down strengthens the whole body: improves blood circulate, prevents arthritis, joint ache, relieves fatigue, anxiety and stress.

Chinese foot rubdown: the principle of reflexology

Chinese foot massage relieves pressure and invigorates. Ancient enjoy has been gathered over the centuries, and these days it allows within the ones moments at the same time as our toes ache or harm. What is the actual technique? And what want to you comprehend approximately it?

Magic dots

In China, because of the reality that historical times, they are saying: "When a tree grows antique, its root is the primary to grow antique. When someone a long time, his ft are the number one to age.

The top notch homes of Chinese foot rubdown are primarily based at the concepts of reflexology. These ideas have been perfected over numerous thousand years via adepts and practitioners of conventional Chinese remedy.

According to these requirements, there are more than 60 factors on the human foot, every of which corresponds to a selected organ or a part of the frame. What does it imply: the country of the foot is a shape of replicate reflecting the internal nation of human organs.

Stimulation of reflex points by way of the usage of manner of urgent them makes it possible to acquire the effect of rest, relieving tension, supporting the body combat ailments, and resisting ailments. But it's far properly well well worth noting one by one: the healing impact of foot rub down need to no longer be exaggerated. This is a extremely good way to take care of your health. But that is a methods from a panacea for all ailments!

Technique

Before the rubdown, it's miles useful to perform one extra and truly quality technique. Namely, to immerse the toes in a basin with a aromatic combination of medicinal herbs that have an amazingly calming effect. This will actually loosen up and set you up for the upcoming rub down.

The technique of Chinese foot massage is numerous, it includes techniques: stress, stroking, rubbing, and vibration. After drying your feet, the masseur will start to paintings with simply considered one of them, wrapping the other in a towel to keep away from cooling and dropping the impact of the recovery bath.

Chapter 28: Optimization Of The Body's Work And Recuperation Impact

Chinese foot rub down method is pretty painful. The masseur applies stress due to the fact best in this case it is possible to spark off and stimulate the critical elements.

And regardless of this, foot rubdown brings pleasure. After the very first consultation, an extraordinary surge of strength is felt. Proven through plenty of years of revel in in historical Chinese remedy.

Chinese rubdown does now not goal to purpose ache. The number one and only goal is to optimize the paintings of the complete organism and the healing effect on the affected or weakened factors of the body. Massage, like numerous remedy, has some of contraindications. Therefore, a preliminary consultation with a scientific health practitioner will not be superfluous.

And in reality found in all corners of the world: after one session with a real Chinese massage expert, your satisfied legs will truly go back you to this professional and to the consequences of his magical way greater than as quickly as.

Foot reflexology: the wonders of a ten-minute rubdown

Foot rubdown is a very top notch method, in particular if your ft are inside the arms of a specialist who is privy to precisely what he is doing. In addition, there are numerous points on the foot which might be associated with numerous elements of the body, and massaging those factors can deliver remedy from pain and relieve exceptional unpleasant signs that stand up in considered one of a type areas of the frame. Reflexology is a workout extensively used in some unspecified time within the destiny of the world, with which you can get rid of numerous styles of issues. Today estet-portal.Com will will let you recognize why foot reflexology is a easy and effective manner to decorate your fitness.

Foot reflexology: long-awaited relaxation for the entire body

The first indeniable advantage of foot reflexology is its potential to loosen up a person and make him forget about about strain. And for folks that spend the entire day on their toes, a foot rubdown is as essential as an middle of the night bathe. Such a massage will assist to easy the direction of strength float and relieve fatigue.

Just five-10 minutes of a smooth and useful massage with crucial oil, which you may choose out out consistent together with your preference and temper, and you may revel in a whole lot better. Foot rubdown with oils may be performed independently, focusing for your feelings.

Foot reflexology - rub down to decorate sleep

If you do a foot rubdown earlier than mattress, it's thrilling effect will assist you fall asleep faster and make your sleep greater restful. Improving blood waft and a laugh the nerves are the quality manner to lighten up at night time.

To benefit a relaxing and fun effect of rubdown, you need to attention at the "foot pad" and the big toe. Allocate at least a minute to rub down the huge toe of every foot, after which rubdown the soles of the toes for each different 10 minutes. This rubdown will be the most beneficial for sleep.

Pain remedy with foot reflexology

There are some of pain situations that can be dealt with with foot reflexology, collectively with pain because of gout, a very painful form of arthritis. Also inside the listing of such pains may be covered:

pain in the neck;

backache;

headache and migraine, and so forth.

Massaging your feet and joints will help relieve neck pain - and this one in just five minutes!

Ankle massage will assist relieve redness and swelling within the region, further to assist lessen headaches and migraines.

Massage of the outer a part of the talus and the Achilles tendon can relieve ache inside the again and hips.

Massaging the arch of the foot can assist relieve pain inside the higher yet again.

Improving blood movement and a surge of power - bonuses of foot reflexology.

If you need to sit down all day at paintings, especially if you positioned on tight jeans and/or like to sit down down circulate-legged, your blood flow into is disrupted. Also, uncomfortable (narrow) shoes make a contribution to the violation of blood motion.

A 10-minute foot reflexology treatment will permit your cells to get sufficient oxygen, so you will sense a real surge of strength. And, importantly, this foot rubdown allows save you the improvement of varicose veins.

Let's recalls that the terrific impact of foot reflexology can be received by using the use of manner of trusting a expert. However, self-rub down of the ft is likewise particular as a safety measure: it permits to alleviate leg fatigue, enhance blood movement, save you varicose veins and clearly flawlessly loosen up you in advance than going to mattress. If you need to make foot reflexology an addition to the precept treatment plan for any disorder, it is higher to are in search of for expert assist or research from a consultant.

Self-Healing Reflexology 10 Steps

This hand reflexology manual consists of ten essential steps for enjoyable self-recuperation.

Step 1 pinching pointers (Squeeze your fingertips and thumb)

Start a relaxing reflexology remedy with a 10 minute hand gripping the pointers of each finger and the thumb of your proper hand. Flip over and repeat this technique for your left hand. The stress at the fingers must be corporation but no longer painful. A few seconds for every fingertip.

Step 2 Pinched aspects of the fingertips (Squeeze the rims of your fingertips and thumb)

After squeezing the tops and bottoms of your fingers and the guidelines of your thumb, skip decrease once more to each tip and squeeze them once more, this time squeezing from side to side. Again, press down, a touch discomfort is right enough. But it is crucial not to harm your self.

Step three Vigorous finger rubbing (Energetic)

Combine steps three and 4 by the use of using rubbing the pinnacle and backside (pictured above) and also rubbing the sides (pictured in step four) of every finger and thumb. Rub vigorously from side to side from base to tip.

Step 4 More energetic rubbing of fingers (Rub the edges of your thumb and hands from base to tip)

Combine steps 3 and four with the aid of the use of way of rubbing the pinnacle and bottom (pictured in step three) and moreover rubbing the perimeters (pictured above) of every finger and thumb. Rub vigorously backward and forward from base to tip.

Step 5 Finger drag (Pull firmly on every finger and thumb)

Grab each finger (and thumb) at the bottom and pull firmly. Let your cope with loosen barely, grade by grade transferring it from the bottom to the pinnacle until your finger is without a doubt out of your hand.

Step 6 Squeeze and pull the webbed location among your arms (Constricted webbed regions among palms)

With your thumb and forefinger, firmly draw near the webbed vicinity between the thumb and forefinger of the other hand. Holding firmly, lightly tug at the pores and pores and skin till the fleshy internet is pulled away from your arms. Repeat this approach for the webbed areas on all arms.

Step 7 Massaging the higher arm with the thumb (Massage the higher a part of the hand with the thumb)

Place your palm in the palm of your loose hand. Use your thumb to rub down the decrease again of your hand. At first, slowly manage the joints and amongst them. Continue massaging every region at the lower returned of your hand together with your thumb.

Step 8 Inner Wrist Massage (Massage Inner Wrist)

Gently fold your wrist in conjunction with your unfastened hand. Use your thumb to massage your internal wrist. This is a mainly soothing rubdown for those who frequently use their wrists in repetitive motions (like mice).

Chapter 29: What Is Acupuncture And Is It Beneficial

Acupuncture is one of the branches of possibility remedy. It is regularly criticized with the aid of manner of adherents of the proof-primarily based clearly approach, consistent with which healing and preventive measures want to be applied first-rate after their effectiveness has been showed with the beneficial aid of medical studies. Nevertheless, the decision for for the services of acupuncturists has been growing in modern-day years, scientists from maximum vital universities like Yale urge no longer to desert remedy truely because of the reality its mechanism is not however completely understood, and all people has heard approximately the analgesic effect of "needles" at the least as soon as from those laid low with arthritis older cherished ones.

We determined to apprehend - as a protracted manner as possible - the person of acupuncture, consulted with supporters and critics of the path, and determined out whether or no longer or now not it modified into actually properly worth attempting this method in any respect.

A resident of the put up-Soviet location, likely, is more familiar with the term "reflexotherapy" - the impact on positive components of the frame with arms, needles, and special devices. Both reflexology and acupuncture on my own are big workout techniques that trade in gear and techniques of influencing lively elements of the frame. In accordance with the philosophy of Eastern treatment (and without philosophy, there is nowhere), those factors aren't positioned randomly, but alongside the meridian channels thru which the essential power qi flows. Qi is one of the important ideas in Chinese lifestyle and alternative remedy, which migrated from there, as an instance, to the New Age: adherents of Chinese philosophy take delivery of as genuine with that it permeates no longer simplest the human frame but the complete worldwide.

www.ingramcontent.com/pod-product-compliance
Lightning Source LLC
Chambersburg PA
CBHW051728020426
42333CB00014B/1201